LIFESTRUCK

Finding Your Best Self <u>Before</u> You Grow Up

PUBLISHED THROUGH LULU ENTERPRISES

3131 RCD CENTER-SUITE 210

MORRISVILLE NC 27560

USA

WWW.LULU.COM

LIFESTRUCK

TABLE OF CONTENTS

AUTHOR BIOGRAPHY

The author is 59 years old and resides in Calgary, Alberta Canada.

Inspired by the Montreal Olympic Games in 1976, the author gave up smoking, a poor diet, and an overall unhealthy way of life and embraced a life of fitness through running. The initial goal was to complete a marathon, and in the spring of 1977 that goal was realized in less than a year when he crossed the finish line of the Calgary Marathon.

Many more marathons and two-fifty mile ultra-marathons followed. After witnessing the 1982 Hawaii Ironman triathlon on ABC Television, the author set his sights on yet another distant finish line and spent a year learning how to swim. In 1984, he crossed the Ironman finish line in Kona.

Entry in 13 more Ironman races followed over the years. After almost three decades of endurance sports, the author created the website "Ironstruck.ca" in the hopes of inspiring and motivating others to become more than they ever thought possible through improved health by way of sound nutrition and a lifestyle of fitness. As of this writing Ironstruck.ca sees visitors from an average of 56 countries a month. Many people around the world have embraced Ironstruck and have used it as a guide to reach their own personal finish line and in the process adopt a better way of life.

Two books were to follow in the path of Ironstruck the website. The first book was Ironstruck ... The Ironman Triathlon Journey, and the second was Ironstruck? 500 Ironman Triathlon Questions and Answers.

Both publications have been very well received by the triathlon world.

INTRODUCTION

As I look back over the past three decades, I can't help but marvel at the course my life has taken. Had it not been for a few events that sparked something within me to take my life in a new direction, I would not be writing this book for you today.

Like most of today's adults, the path my life followed was greatly influenced by what happened back in junior high and high school.

Even though over 4 decades have passed since my school years, I can still remember those days with a clarity that, to me, speaks volumes about the impact those years had on my life.

I can remember the urgency of trying to fit in, of trying to find somewhere to belong. I remember how everyone tried to find a group that would accept them. There were the smart kids who gravitated toward each other, the ethnic groups, and the beautiful people who had the looks and all the latest clothes. Then of course there were those fortunate ones who were skilled and athletic enough to make it on one of the school sports teams. There were even those who belonged to more than one group, and then there were those who couldn't seem to fit in anywhere.

I was one of those who struggled to fit in. I came from a broken family and there was never the money to keep up with the image portrayed by the kids who came from a more stable home environment. I wanted desperately to be on the school teams but was never quite able to make it.

There was a very short window of opportunity when it came to being chosen for a team. Forty kids might try out for the basketball team and the coach had to pick 12 or so of the best. It was the same in all the school sports. It was a devastating blow to my confidence and sense of self-worth once I realized I was never going to be quite good enough. Even though many years have passed since I walked the halls of my school, I have a feeling that it's not all that much different now.

Those who can't seem to fit in anywhere tend to attract others who are pretty much in the same boat. Yes, there is even a group for kids who can't find a group. I call them "fringe groups." I think the guys I hung out with all pretty much considered themselves losers. In place of the sports I wanted to take up, I took up smoking and drinking and simply just "hanging around" looking for something to fill in the time. The school years that should have been a special time in my life were sad and something I just had to withstand. All the same, I consider myself fortunate that drugs were not a big thing back then or the consequences might have been a lot worse.

Regardless, the seeds that were planted in those high school years took root and once I left school behind, not much changed. I was 28 years old before something moved me enough to make me realize that I had the ability to make changes in my life. It was then that I figured out that I could still be the athlete I had wanted to be back in high school. I ditched the cigarettes and beer and took up running. It was a few years after my lifestyle of fitness began when I saw my first triathlon on T.V. and realized that I had found the sport for me. I couldn't swim a stroke at the time, but I didn't care. I would learn. I was going to be in that race I saw on T.V. I was going to be a triathlete.

Two years later I found myself in Kona, Hawaii. I was entered in what was considered one of the toughest races in the world at the time. There I was making the turn for home in the 3.8 km swim leg of the Hawaii Ironman. Who would ever have imagined it possible? Me, the kid who could never make the team and who just two years before couldn't swim a single stroke. Some 14 hours later I crossed the finish line of what has become the "mother" of all triathlons. My life was never the same again.

I ended up having a running and triathlon career that lasted almost 3 decades. I went on to build a website that would inspire others to test the boundaries of their ability on so many levels. All that was missing was a name for my site. I chose the name "Ironstruck." I wanted a word to define the moment when a person comes to the realization that there is more to life than being a spectator. A word that would define that moment when they see something, hear something, or read something that inspires them to change the course of their lives.

I wrote two "Ironstruck" books as well that I hoped would help adults find their way to a healthier more fulfilling way of life and hopefully motivate them and instill confidence in them.

I was shocked when I realized just how many adults were in need of something to inspire them to make a positive change. I don't mean just in Canada or North America. I mean around the world. There are just so many adults who lack confidence in their own ability. Adults who have poor diets, poor physical conditioning, and lives that seem to be begging for a change in direction.

I'm glad to say that "Ironstruck" has moved many people to challenge themselves and make changes in the way they live their lives.

I will always believe that the most important thing to do first if you want to be successful in this world is to embrace a healthy lifestyle. In the long run, it won't really matter how rich you are, how smart you are, or how lofty your station in life. If you don't have control of your physical health and well-being, material success can quickly become insignificant.

The more I thought about it, the more I realized that it's in the school years where inspiration and motivation are most needed. Those are the formative school years that can easily decide the happiness, health and success that you carry into adulthood. Those are the years that have the most impact toward deciding the direction your life will take. Far too often, chance can have a dramatic effect on your self-esteem, health, and confidence.

It can be as simple as trying out for a team in your first year of high school and not making it. Maybe you even try 2 or 3 times to make different teams but just don't seem to be quite good enough. After a while, you just give up and accept your fate. You might even start to doubt your own ability and begin to dread going to Phys ed classes. Your fitness suffers as you look for different avenues to vent all your pent up youthful energy.

You might turn to smoking, drugs, drinking, excessive eating, or even closing yourself in your room for hours on end as you lose yourself in computer games and chat rooms. Poor diet might eventually lead to weight problems or eating disorders, and ultimately, poor health. It seems that your life is spinning out of control as your self-esteem reaches a new low.

It doesn't have to be that way.

I truly believe that participation in sports and a healthy diet are vital for students as they prepare for their journey into adulthood. Success in reaching whatever athletic goals you set for yourself and attaining the body image you are comfortable with through exercise and healthy eating equates into a sense of well-being and increased self-esteem that can ultimately be the perfect springboard toward becoming a vibrant, healthy, and confident adult.

So how do you find your sport? If you can't make a team in school, what do you do? What do you do for fitness? Where do you turn?

A really great starting point might be to become a triathlete. You can become a member of the fastest growing sport in the world. There is a reason why triathlon is being so widely accepted. It's mainly because it's a sport for *everyone*. You don't *have to* compete against anyone. You don't *have to* make a team. If you can't swim, then you can take lessons and learn how. Almost everyone knows how to ride a bike. Most likely you can already walk fast or run a little. Once you can do all three disciplines you are well on your way to becoming a triathlete. The best part is, it's not necessary to have an athletic background in order to take the sport up. The most important requirement is to have a passion for what you are doing and the will to make a change.

You have the power within you to make changes and do amazing things with your life. It's right at your fingertips, and maybe I can help you unleash that power and discover for yourself just how special and dynamic you really are.

Maybe this book will be the catalyst for achieving the "new, improved" you. Once you get out there and find out how great it feels to be fit and strong, it may lead you to another sport that is even more perfect for you. Maybe you will develop a passion for running or swimming. Maybe the confidence and fitness you gain from being a triathlete will help you make that soccer team or volleyball team you always wanted to be a part of. It's not so much the sport you choose as it is embracing fitness with spirit and enthusiasm as a way of life. The important thing is to find your groove and to begin your transformation to a healthier way of living every single day.

I have called this book LIFESTRUCK. It's all about embracing the power you have within you to control the course of your life and unleashing the ability within you to reach levels of physical fitness, sound health, and academic standing you never thought possible.

> Lifestruck is about building a solid foundation that will stay with you and support you for all the days of your life.

- ➢ Lifestruck is about having fun, being healthy, and being strong. It is about building your confidence and self-esteem through sports inspired fitness and a healthy diet and carrying it over into all aspects of your life.

- ➢ Lifestruck is about realizing there indeed is "a better way."

You are the hope of the future. It is **you** who will inherit this world. There are many challenges ahead as you evolve into adulthood, but at the same time I'm optimistic that you have what it takes to make positive changes and be up for the challenge.

In this book I will discuss some of the problems some of you may well be dealing with right now. I will also try and provide you with some insight into healthy eating and how fitness through sports and a sound diet are so closely linked and how they can combine to make you healthier, stronger and more confident as you make your way in this world.

I will also give you a bit of insight into triathlon and just why it might be the sport that will help turn your life around.

I'm writing this book for you, not as a doctor, teacher, coach or professional of any sort, but rather as an adult who remembers very well the impact the teenage years can have on the rest of your life.

I am writing this book as an amateur athlete with a career spanning three decades that involved competing in over 35 marathons, 14 Ironman triathlons, 2 50-mile road races, and over 100 other races of varying distances.

Most of all I am writing this book for you from personal experience and years of experimenting with eating properly combined with a lifestyle of fitness. That, along with my 40 year career in the retail grocery industry, will give you some unique insight into the world of food and what has brought us, and more importantly, *you*, to where we find ourselves today.

I hope with all my heart that this book will encourage you and help you to understand that you are never too young to take charge of your life. I hope it will start you on a journey of self-discovery that will result in your becoming a confident, healthy, and well adjusted adult. Take a leap of faith, believe in yourself, never give up, and soon you will discover just how much you are capable of on so many levels.

You will be amazed. You will be thrilled.

You will be "Lifestruck."

Chapter One

I'M OVERWEIGHT. IS IT TOO LATE FOR ME? *

You are truly magnificent.

You just don't realize it.

You look in the mirror and see a lump of coal instead of the sparkling diamond you have the power to become. The more time that passes, the harder it is to see yourself as much more than just another fat kid in school. Trust me, you are not alone. Obesity in youth is increasing at an astounding rate in North American schools. This impacts all aspects of your life and poor nutrition habits in school can cause serious health problems in adulthood. It's also a well known fact that your nutrition and fitness habits can dramatically influence how you perform academically.

It might even seem to you that you are doomed and condemned to your lot in life and there is no getting away from it. That is so far from the truth.

You are a miracle of creation, and it's up to you to take full advantage of the gift of life and all the possibilities that are yours for the taking. There is no need to accept less than your full potential. Maybe settling for less seems like the easiest way out, but keep in mind that anything worth having is worth sacrificing and working for. Often the road you will travel over the adult years of your life is decided in your school years. That's why it's so important to realize that even as a young adult it's important to accept responsibility for yourself and take charge of your life.

What you see in the mirror is what your past has led you to. Regardless of whether it's a poor diet, lack of nutritional knowledge, family problems, or low self-esteem that has brought you to where you are at this point in your life, it's important to remember that it's *in the past*.

Once you understand and accept that, then every single minute in front of you provides an opportunity to change the direction you are going. It's almost like there will always be a door in front of you waiting to be opened. Your future will always be yours to change. Just open the door and on the other side you will find a new path you can choose to follow. It takes courage, self-discipline, and passion, but if it's in your heart to change, you will succeed. It's your life and it's important that you take control of it. It's time to be responsible. It's time to stop looking for someone or something to blame.

More than anything, it's time for action. Ultimately your destiny is in your hands, and the course of your life decades from now could very well be decided by the decisions you make in your school years.

I truly believe that the most important change to make first is a physical one. Your health must come first above all else. That means getting yourself fit. It means challenging your body physically to improve, and it means fueling your body properly.

Your body does everything in its power to react to what you demand of it. If you work your muscles and challenge them, your body responds by making them toned and strong. If you have a sound diet, you will be helping your body do its work. If you never exercise and live on junk food, your body will still do its best to help you make it through the day, but it will be over-worked and stressed. A poor diet will constrict your arteries and force your heart to work harder to keep you functioning.

Imagine drinking water through a straw. It's fairly easy to draw the water up the straw to your mouth. Now imagine if the straw has an opening only half the size. You have to work a lot harder to make the water flow.

That's pretty much what happens when your arteries become clogged because of poor diet and lack of conditioning. Your heart has to work much harder to ensure that blood flows to where it is needed in your body. That's why you might struggle for breath by simply walking up a flight of stairs. You can almost hear the pounding in your chest of your heart working hard trying to get you where you want to go.

If you combine a good healthy diet with a commitment to a higher level of fitness, you will see dramatic changes in your body. Although it might take a year or two to project the healthy body image you would like to portray, you will begin to notice changes very quickly once you take action and set out on your journey of self-discovery. Before you know it, you will go from fat to fit and from weak to strong. Each milestone you reach and each obstacle you overcome will give you even more encouragement to keep pressing forward, ever forward.

Give yourself a chance and I can almost guarantee that one day in the not too distant future you will look in that same mirror in complete awe at the reflection you see. That moment is so worth striving for, because it will change your life forever. You will have a new understanding of just how much you are truly capable of on so many levels.

Once you make a commitment to becoming fit, strong, and healthy in your body, the rest of the uniqueness that defines who you are will begin to shine through as well. The sparkling diamond that you truly are has always been there just waiting for the day when you buff it up and let it glow for all the world to see.

Start today. Release the power you have within and let your spirit sing.

Chapter Two

* THE PERFECT BODY *

Everyone wants to be accepted. Everyone wants to fit in. Everyone wants to appear desirable to others. Far too often, however, teens will push the envelope and go to extremes to attain what they see as the perfect body image. For some teens, usually girls, it can seem like a never ending battle to achieve and maintain their idea of physical perfection. Over the past few decades the "thinner is better" notion has somehow manifested itself on young adult and adult women. Crash diets and exercising far too much are a few of the methods used to achieve that look. It's a recipe for disaster.

Having a weight problem doesn't just mean being overweight; it can mean being far too underweight as well. I mean the kind of underweight caused by eating disorders that can easily result in illness and even spending time in the hospital.

It's a sad fact that eating disorders among teenage girls is on the rise in North America. In a 2004 survey of girls 10-14, almost 30% claimed to be on a diet. Do you obsess about your weight? Do you have dizzy spells? Do you have a short attention span in school? Do you sometimes just feel really crappy for no apparent reason? These are all warning signs, and it's imperative that you talk to someone about it. Talk to your parents or your family doctor or a school counselor or teacher, but talk to someone.

The other day I read something interesting in an entertainment magazine. The discussion was about two Hollywood actresses and how thin they were. Someone made the comment "you know, I've never actually seen either of them eat anything."

They both weighed around 90 pounds (40kg) and were almost skeletal, and yet obviously perceived themselves as being glamorous. It's almost as if they just can't get thin enough. It doesn't take a professional to figure out that some sort of emotional and self-esteem issues must be part of the problem.

Our bodies are not made to function without nourishment. Sure you will lose weight if you simply quit eating, but eventually your body will shut down because it just can't do its best work without proper fuel in the way of wholesome food. You are actually forcing your body to feed on itself. Your muscles will stop growing and developing, and most of the essential systems in your body will suffer and cease to work properly. You are leaving your body no way to fight off disease. There are numerous studies that have shown that eating disorders can cause heart, liver, and kidney problems.

Fat has many important functions. Your body needs fat as a padding to protect vital organs. Fat is also part of the membrane in almost every cell in your body including nerve, brain, and skin cells. It's also important as protection from the cold.

There is another more natural alternative you can choose that will have a positive impact on your health, vitality, and the body image you project. It's no secret that girls who choose healthy nutrition choices and are physically fit have high self-esteem. That usually results in being more popular and more likely to do better academically in school. There is a huge difference between being physically fit and eating smart and exercising and starving yourself until you feel like passing out. Your goal might be to make yourself look more desirable, but ultimately you will deprive yourself of the vitality that comes with giving your body the basic raw materials of nutrition and fitness it needs to ensure you look and feel your best.

I recall seeing the cover of a magazine a few months before the Olympics. It featured three of the women who would be competing for Canada in Beijing. One was a swimmer, one was a runner, and one was a gymnast. They looked stunning. Their hair had an amazing shine to it and their eyes were bright and clear. They all had such a healthy glow and even the way they smiled had a hint of the confidence they had in themselves.

Do you think for a minute that they starved themselves to look so beautiful? Do you think they have trouble getting a date? Do you think for one moment they struggle with self-esteem? Not in this lifetime. You can bet they ate like troopers in order to provide the fuel they needed to sustain their high level of fitness. It is within your reach to attain that same level of well-being. The rewards of healthy living are not reserved just for world class athletes. It is there for you as well and all you have to do is reach out and take it.

If you feed your body properly, you will be providing a cleaner burning fuel for it to burn. A sensible exercise and fitness plan coupled with a sound diet to replace what you burn is the way to a truly spectacular new you.

If you give your body a fair chance, it will soon begin to respond to what you are asking of it. If you do your part by giving it the fuel it needs to perform at peak efficiency, it will reward you by creating an amazingly healthy body image that will bring with it renewed confidence, superior health, and the best kind of self-esteem that you will carry with you for the rest of your life.

You will be amazed at the shine in your hair, the light in your eyes, and the bounce in your step if you choose a healthier path to achieve a body image you will be proud of.

Chapter Three

* I DON'T FIT IN *

Let me guess. You could never imagine yourself making a school team. You cringe whenever you have to do anything fitness related in school. It's really tough to make friends, and just being in school every day is a challenge as you struggle to find just where you fit in.

Really, nothing has changed much from the time I was in high school. Every school no matter where it happens to be probably has about the same general make-up. It seems that just days into the high school year everyone is in a scramble to belong somewhere.

It never fails.

There will be the ones who are good at sports and there will be the really bright kids who will hang out with other bright kids.

Then there is always an "in" crowd who are fortunate enough to be able to wear all the latest clothes and have all the latest toys.

Then there is always that "fringe" group.

That was my high school group. You never worried much about keeping up with the latest in fashion because your family just never had any money. You would try out for some school teams and never quite make it. Your grades are okay but not spectacular. So it's only natural to gravitate towards others who are much like yourself. You find ways to rebel. Back in the day we would sit in a local restaurant and smoke. On the weekends we would drink. High school was just something to endure and not something to look forward to.

It's an inescapable fact that the path you follow in high school might well chart the direction your future will take for many years after. Perhaps even for the rest of your life.

Yet if you really think about it, even with all the groups you find in pretty well every school in the world, there are always those remarkable kids who seem to fit in with anyone. They have a certain aura about them. They are self-confident and so sure of themselves. They are kind and look down on no one. They never get bullied. They are good in sports and do well academically. They never have problems when it comes to dating. Others gravitate toward them, so having friends is never a problem. They have set their sights on the direction they want to go with their lives and are running with it.

In short, they believe in themselves. They seem to have an inner strength that allows them to forge ahead in life without the need to be part of any specific school group in order to build their confidence and sense of belonging. Often these are the kids who end up being the student president or voted "most likely to succeed."

The power to become a confident, self-assured person is within you. Feeling confident in any situation and with anyone begins with feeling good about yourself. The secret is to make positive changes in a few key areas like your fitness and nutrition and learn how to live life with a *passion*. Once you feel good about

33

yourself and the image you portray, your confidence will grow as well and soon **you** will become the person others want to be around and fitting in will no longer be a problem.

It might not be easy to get there, but you can do it and the rewards can last a lifetime.

Chapter Four

I remember going on a field trip back in grade ten (about 43 years ago) when I was a student in a Vancouver high school. Our teacher took us to the head office of a major bank. It was about a six story building and one entire floor was home to their brand new computer. I mean the *entire* floor. I remember how proud they were of their computer and how they wowed us by letting us play tic-tac-toe with it.

We thought that was one smart computer because it couldn't be beat. As soon as you made a move it made its counter move right away. The best anyone could do was tie it. It had two responses at the end of a game. There was no computer screen. There was a printer. It would print out, "it's a tie! or "you lose!" We thought that was so cool. We had no idea. We simply had no idea that we were looking at the forerunner of a technology that would one day sweep across the world. A technology so advanced that it would create billionaires, break down international borders, and completely change the way life would be lived on a day to day basis.

The ability of a computer is stunning. There is no other word for it. It's simply stunning, especially if, like my generation, you lived in this world when they simply never existed.

For most of you reading this book, that's certainly not the case. I saw my first T.V. set when I was 7 years old. By the time you were seven, you were most likely already the overlord of the computer in your home. You could travel to distant lands, learn facts about the world that at one time took weeks or months of research, and figure out in a heartbeat how your dad lost the letter he was working on into a big black pit in the far reaches of megabyte land.

For me that field trip to see my first ever computer was a mere glimpse of what was to come. Little did I know what the future would bring. How could I ever have imagined that one day high school students would have a small computer in their backpack or in their bedroom that would outperform by 1000 times or more the monster that took up an entire floor of a huge office building?

Students of today have access to amazing technology that was unheard of just decades ago. With the click of a mouse you have a wealth of knowledge at your fingertips. You can do research for any school project, or chat with a friend down the block or across the ocean. You can Google pretty well any subject, and thousands of responses will pop up instantly.

Maybe you are one of those who have found a haven and escape from the pressures of school in your computer screen. More than that, maybe it has become an escape from the real world. It's somewhere you can go and not be judged. You know that you can be big, small, fat, skinny, white or black and it won't matter to your computer. It's easy to just lose yourself in computer games. Computer games are great, but are they the best way to utilize what spare time you have left once you spend a day in school, do your homework, and sleep for eight hours?

For a moment, just think about that big computer I told you about that I saw on the school field trip. Why do you think the bank had it built? I'm sure they didn't build it just so they could play tic-tac-toe with it. They had it built to keep a record of their business dealings and their clients. It was built to store information.

Many years ago the main branch of the public library ran a contest. They wanted people to submit a name for their new computer system. They had hundreds of entries. It took me about 15 minutes to come up with the name I was pretty sure had a great chance of winning. That's how long it took me to get to the nearest branch of the library and find a Latin-English translation book.

I looked up the word "knowledge" and there was the Latin translation and winning name staring back at me.

"ROGO." *To store knowledge.*

What a great name. It was short and compact, and what librarian could resist the Latin connection? I sent the name in, and several weeks later I received a letter from the library.

You won't believe this. It really blew me away, but this is what the letter said.

"Thank you so much for submitting the great winning name "ROGO" for our new city wide computer system. We just wanted you to know that the name of our security system is NOGO."

What are the odds? Of course I had no idea about the name of their security system. They must have looked at the name I picked and the name of their security system and just quit opening letters. It was basically pure luck and quite a coincidence.

"ROGO". To store knowledge.

That's what a computer is all about. It's about reaching people and reaching out and touching the world. It's about supplying and obtaining knowledge. Computers are spectacular. Love your computer, but love it for all the right reasons.

What a difference it would make to your health and fitness if you took your weekends and those precious hours you have left in your day after school, homework, and sleeping, and spent more time being physically active. At first it might be a challenge to pull yourself away from your computer and head to the pool for a swim, or for a run around the block, but the fitter you get, the better you will start to feel.

Your body wants to move, be strong, be healthy, and flow in concert with the Universe. It doesn't want to sit idle with the sole function of improving your eye-hand coordination. Physical activity releases endorphins that make you feel really good, and the fitter you get, the better it feels.

Give it a chance.

Give your body a chance. Work with it. Understand it.

Understand what it needs to operate at peak efficiency in all aspects. I can say with all the knowledge and experience I have gained in over 3 decades of striving for the best possible fitness level I could attain that your body will respond if you persist and develop a passion for becoming all you are capable of.

Take control of your nutrition and take control of your fitness. Start to use all of your body. Move. Always move and feel your body respond. Walk, jog, run, swim, or bike. At first it may not be far or fast, but with each passing day you will sense a change taking place. You will begin to feel better. Your body will be rushing to build, tone, and strengthen those muscles that have been dormant for so one. Fat will begin to disappear as it's burned for fuel. Soon your body will be demanding more healthy food to supply the vital nutrients it needs to construct the "new you."

With increased physical activity and a healthier diet you will sleep better and feel better. By choosing a healthier lifestyle you will be making the most of all those hours you used to spend in front of your computer. Each day that you see change and improvement will fuel your enthusiasm even more as you continue on your path to a way of life that will benefit you for all the days of your life. Your self-esteem will grow with each success and soon others will take notice. In time, as you become fitter and happier with the body image you portray to the world, an aura will envelop you. It's an aura of well-being and it will attract others to you. Others will want to be like you. They will want to know your secret.

You will discover that there is no "high" in the world like a natural high. A high that you earn through doing something remarkable that has come from within. Unlike the false highs of drugs, alcohol, and computer games, which are deceptive and fleeting, a natural high is a high that will stay with you for a long, long time.

Sometimes forever.

I experienced that almost a quarter of a century ago. I experienced it when I took on the challenge of the Hawaii Ironman in Kona in 1984 while it was still an event quite new to the world. It was as if in one day I purged all those school years of unhappiness, low self-esteem, and one failure after another in the course of a single day. I went from the depressed kid who could never make a school team to an adult who finally arrived and understood for the first time that most of the limitations we have in life are the ones we impose on ourselves. It took me 35 years to figure it out.

I remember the euphoria of conquering the 3.8 km swim and heading out onto the 180 km bike ride into the oven they called the King K. Highway. The Lava fields, oppressive hot winds, and long hills made muscles scream and want to stop. Still, I was on a mission and there was a finish line in the distance I wanted to cross more than anything. The bike was followed by a full 42.2 km marathon and it was unforgettable. It got to be a battle of will to take every single step.

Never, never will I forget running into Kona and the last kilometer of that long, long day. I was all alone and in a twist of fate there were no other runners around me. It was just over 14 hours since I had set out on the swim and now as I turned the final corner I instinctively knew that my life would never be quite the same again. The final half kilometer to the finish line was lined with thousands of spectators. Night had fallen and four huge spotlights marked the finish line ahead, and I found out later it was the ABC television camera lights.

When I woke up the next morning, I was on an incredible high from what had taken place the day before. The amazing thing is, it never went away. That one experience changed the course of my life forever and has led me to where I am right now, writing this book for you. Even today when I think of that final stretch to the finish line I can hear the crowd, see those bright lights, and taste the salt in the crisp night air as if it all just happened yesterday. Can you say that about your computer game session last week, two days ago, or even yesterday?

Somewhere in your future, there are bright lights and finish lines just waiting for you to arrive. Begin your journey with one small positive step into the world of fitness, and you will be amazed at the power it has to change your life for the better.

Chapter Five

* THE BULLY BLUES *

The cheetah hides in the tall grass and studies the herd. As he creeps closer the herd senses danger and the stampede begins, but already the hunter has picked out his prey. Instinctively he targets the loner who is not quite as strong and fast as the others and just can't keep up. As he closes in, the predator can sense the fear emanating from his prey ,and it spurs him on with renewed confidence as he closes in for the kill.

It sort of reminds me of the bully in school who sensed right away that I was the one to pick on. In truth, it was almost like I and a few others were targeted from the very beginning. I guess we must have stood out from the rest of the herd and looked like easy targets.

In reality, bullies are nothing more than predators who go after the weak and defenseless. Like the cheetah in the tall grass, school bullies can sense your fear and uncertainty. Usually the weak ones are not just weak physically, but also have very low self-esteem as well and just don't have very much confidence in themselves. When you lack self-confidence it's pretty difficult to find the courage to stand up for yourself.

When I think back, it seemed there were two critical times when the bullying was the worst. Those times were the first year of junior high school and then again when I started high school. It seems to make sense now, because those are two major stepping stones in the school years and it tends to put extra pressure on some students to assert themselves and find their place in the big scheme of things.

In reality, your average bully doesn't have a much better self-image than the people he targets, and in his own way, he is looking for a way to fit in and gain some sort of recognition. As misguided as their motives are, it seems to be the only thing they can think of doing to try and build up their self-esteem. I distinctly remember that by the time grades eleven and twelve rolled around the bullying in general had pretty well stopped.

Either the bullies never made it that far in school or they had a change in attitude for some reason. More likely it was because they finally matured and realized just how ridiculous they were making themselves look.

There is even cyber bullying now. To me it's just an indication of exactly the type of people bullies are. If the best they can do is hide behind the anonymity of a computer screen, then I would assume all their other attention-getting methods aren't working all that well. Cyber bullying is nothing more than an extension of the bullying that goes on at school. Nothing anyone says or does can bother you unless you let it.

Unfortunately you were born into an age where technology is a big part of your life and it's very difficult not to be seriously upset if someone says something nasty about you online. After all it's computers, cell-phones, laptops, and text messaging that you use to plug into your world. To you it's like being ridiculed in front of everyone. In reality, probably not as many people as you might think actually see it or take it seriously.

However, there are steps you can take to help prevent or to deal with online bullying.

First of all, be cautious when giving out any of your online contact information. Give potential friends time to prove themselves before allowing them to much access to your life. You will have many *acquaintances* in school, but very few true *friends*. There's a big difference between the two. Just giving your cell phone number to the wrong person can open you up to a barrage of unwanted text messages. Be sure you can trust the people you give it to, and make sure they understand to keep it to themselves.

It's best not to engage in online communication with a bully. All that does is let them know they are getting to you and encourages them to keep it up. Most chat sites, etc. give you the ability to block others from contacting you. Do this as soon as possible.

Also, be sure to print off copies of the offending material in case it persists and becomes serious enough that authorities might have to step in. Some bullies might not realize it, but it can be considered a criminal offense to attack someone on the Internet.

Be sure to let your parents know. Your first reaction might be to keep it to yourself because you might lose your computer privileges, but chances are your parents are not going to place blame on you and together you can work out a strategy to deal with the problem. Believe me, you will feel much better if you talk with someone about cyber bullying. Yes, you might be better with computers than your parents, but they will have a better knowledge of safety issues and what goes on out in the world around you.

It doesn't matter if you are being bullied in person or online, it can be a fearful thing to deal with. I can remember the days when I actually feared going to school. I just didn't have the confidence to stand up for myself, and bullies can sense that in a heartbeat.

One day the same bully picked on me once too often. I simply wasn't willing to take any more. I don't even know for sure what happened next, but instead of being fearful I became a bit angry and stood up to him. It was the first time I had ever reacted to the bully in that way. I had simply had enough and made sure that was the message he got.

That was the last time that he ever bothered me. Like the cheetah, he just went after a prey that was weaker and didn't want to bother with someone who was strong in any way and who would give him problems.

Here are a few things you should remember that I hope will help you deal with bullying.

First of all, you should never start trouble or instigate a fight. At all costs you should avoid conflict. If you can't, then sometimes it's necessary to make a "show of force." It doesn't necessarily mean hitting anyone or getting physical. It just means that you stand up to them and show them that you will defend yourself if necessary. Often that's the only thing a bully will understand. You may be deathly afraid, but often just sending the message that you won't be putting up with their bullying anymore could well bring an end to your problem. Just be sure that you evaluate the situation carefully and pick the right spot. For instance it's far better if you are in or around the school so teachers can intervene if necessary.

Also, instead of responding to them and playing their game when they make threats, try speaking a truth they can't dispute. For instance, "I don't want to fight with you." I want to get along with you." "I would sooner be your friend." Make every effort you can to reason with them without letting the bully draw you into a confrontational dialogue.

Bullying doesn't go on forever. Try not to let it get you down by thinking that your whole life will be like this. It won't. The older you get, the more options you will have when it comes to avoiding the bullies. It just seems that in school you have no choice but to deal with it.

There are four short words from the bible that have helped me through many difficult times in my life. You might want to remember them.

"This too shall pass."

At times life can be very trying. No matter how bad things seem, don't ever give up on yourself and think for a minute that things will never get better. *All* things pass. Time is a great healer. Situations change, people change and time marches on. Bullies get kicked out of school, avoid you because they know you just won't put up with them anymore, or for some reason change their ways. One way or the other it will end.

Absolutely the best thing you can do is work on your confidence and self-esteem by dedicating yourself to becoming stronger and healthier in body and mind.

I can't stress enough how it will help you so much in every aspect of your life. Become the best you can be with what you have and for your entire life you will be a force to be reckoned with.

Chapter Six

SECOND CHANCES

You might have the impression that you've made such of a mess of your life already that it's just too late for you to change the path you are on. Maybe you already have drinking, drug, or smoking addictions that seem insurmountable. Maybe you've already been in trouble with the law. Regardless of what has brought you to this point in your life, you are pretty certain that most of the people who know you will doubt you and your ability to change.

Yes, at times it can be a very unforgiving world, and often you might get the feeling that others have given up on you as they continue to move forward and excel and you fall by the roadside of life. However the image you portray to others is of your own making and if that image is not so great, then it's up to you to change your life in such a way that others can't help but see you in a new light.

You might just be in for a big surprise.

People notice things. So many people want the underdog to succeed. Even if they don't come right out and say it, they can't help but notice if your life suddenly begins to take on a new direction. They might wonder what's happening. They might think "this will never last" or most likely they will be on your side and will take a wait and see attitude. Real friends and family may even give you their full support from the very beginning and never lose faith in you as they see you make the attempt to turn your life around.

Often people who fail to show support and are all to quick to desert you in your darkest hour are not the type of people you want to surround yourself with anyway. You will know soon enough where true loyalty lies and who indeed is a friend worth having.

Here are a couple of examples of what I mean.

When Lance Armstrong lay fighting for his life against cancer and was a mere shadow of himself as he was at death's door, there were sponsors that dropped him like a hot potato. Their reasoning was that he was never going to make any money for them in his condition so it was best to simply sever all ties with him and look for another star to make them rich.

Then there was the sponsor who came in and said to Lance, "no matter what happens, we will be here for you. We will never desert you and we will fight this battle together."

They looked far past seeing Lance as a client, but rather saw him as a person fighting for another chance at life.

So who do you think was rewarded when Lance went on to win his battle against cancer and became one of the world's greatest cyclists by winning the Tour D' France over and over again?

If you are reading this book and have doubts about turning your life around, you should also know this story about Canadian equestrian Eric Lamaze.

The 40-year-old was banned from the sport of equestrianism three different times. On one occasion it was for 4 years and the other two times it was for life. He was accused of drug use. The really sad part was how quick the upper echelons of the horse set were to jump to conclusions and in doing so give the impression that "he is not one of us." In all those years he never was truly accepted by them.

He was dropped from the Canadian team just prior to the 1996 Olympics and banned from the sport for 4 years. The ban was later reduced because it was proven that the cocaine was not taken for competitive advantage. Four years passed and he was banned for life after testing positive for the stimulant ephedrine. According to an article in the Globe and Mail, "the positive test results were from a supplement called Diet Pep that Lamaze had been using for years with no problem, but the makers had changed the ingredients without changing the label." As a result the lifetime ban was dropped.

Just weeks later, Lamaze tested positive for cocaine once again and was again banned for life. Mr. Danson, his lawyer and good friend, argued that Eric had been in a spiral of depression since being banned from the Olympic Games in Sydney through no fault of his own. Things got so bad that Eric was actually in a suicidal state by this time. Once again the ban was lifted, but still Eric never got to compete in the Olympics and even though he worked his way back onto the Canadian team the next year, the horse set still kept him at arms length.

Finally the true story of the life of Eric Lamaze came to light. He was first exposed to cocaine by his mother who was addicted to the drug while pregnant. Even as a baby, he was given the drug by his mother. He never knew who his father was, and he was eventually raised by an alcoholic grandmother.

How can it be such a surprise that he developed a drug abuse problem as a teenager? Things were so bad, Eric dropped out of school in grade 7.

Despite these three major setbacks to his career, Eric still fought on and quit cocaine on his own. For a decade he rebuilt his life and stayed clean and became a trainer and a coach. Many experts were to claim later that most people would have been dead or complete drug addicts, but despite everything, Eric Lamaze never gave up. All he ever wanted was that second chance to prove himself.

In reality he was never cheating, but was the victim of circumstances that began before he took his very first breath in this world. Yet despite that, so many were quick to give up on him. All except people like his friend and sports lawyer who had nothing but admiration for the strength and character it took for Eric to fight his way back to the top as he sought redemption and a chance to repay Canada for the embarrassment he felt he had caused his country.

That opportunity was to come in Beijing, China when Eric Lamaze was sitting on his horse Hickstead, awaiting the start of his ride for the medals in the 2008 Olympic Games. What could he have been thinking as his life had led him to this point in time? All that was in his past, and all the doubters and nay sayers were soon to be silenced as Eric Lamaze and Hickstead were sensational and won the Gold medal for Canada.

Later Eric said to a reporter, "we should never forget the merits of giving a second and third chance to those who are struggling."

So you are a young adult and wonder if there is a second chance in this world for you?

Of course there is. You have your whole life in front of you and have the capability to change the path you are on at any time. What has happened to you is in the past, but the future has yet to unfold. The years ahead of you are a clean slate and what is written on the blackboard of your future is entirely up to you.

Chapter Seven

* WHAT IS A HEALTHY DIET? *

There have been thousands of books written on diets of every description. A lot of what you read probably seems like smoke and mirrors and there's no doubt it can be confusing if you are attempting to make a change for the better in your eating habits. It can be very difficult and often frustrating just trying to find a starting point. Just the fact that so many people are quick to accept the newest fad diet and give it a try is an obvious indication they are not happy with the way they look and feel. The diets that seem to be the most popular at first are the ones that appear to take the least amount of effort. That's why most of them never work and the resulting failure to achieve the desired changes ends up being disheartening and just another blow to already decimated self-esteem.

It takes effort and commitment and the willingness to accept that a wholesale change must be made in the way that food is perceived in order to achieve the desired results. It's important to understand that food is more than a source of instant gratification, but in reality is the very essence of life itself. It doesn't matter if you're a flower, a tree, a bear, or a person; how you blossom and how you grow and live your life are determined for the most part on the nutrients that sustain you.

I suppose in simple terms it would make sense to say that a healthy diet is a diet that provides your body with the necessary nutrients to ensure that you continue to function at optimum levels both physically and mentally.

The problem is, we live in an age where those essential nutrients have become lost in a sea of processed food, sugar substitutes, chemical additives, preservatives, pesticides, fertilizers, fast food, and poor quality fats.

I'm sure you've heard of the basic food groups that include grains, fruits and vegetables, milk and other dairy products, and meat, including fish and chicken. In simpler terms, these food groups provide a blend of carbohydrates, protein, and fat.

At one time it was pretty basic and simple when it came to eating right.

For instance, just think about the first people to ever walk on the face of the earth. What do you think their diet might have consisted of? Most likely they ate meat, fish, roots, eggs, herbs, and berries. Well, how about that! Carbohydrates, protein, and fat and not one jelly-filled donut in sight. So maybe the caveman had it right all along and we are just coming to that realization in North America now. There is no denying that our society faces problems with obesity, eating disorders, and over-all poor eating habits that can often lead to heart disease, diabetes, cancer, insomnia, depression, fatigue, and in some cases, an early death.

So what happened? How did we get to where we are today? If we are so advanced and civilized why does it look like we aren't as smart as a caveman? Where did we go wrong?

For starters, early civilization never had the temptations that bombard you every single day. Their main focus was to eat to survive and stay healthy and strong so they could make it from day to day in a world where it was a challenge to kill animals for food without becoming their main course first. So it was the strong who survived and lived a longer, healthier life. So why should it be any different for you? Wouldn't it make sense to embrace a wholesome way of fueling your body so you can live a long and healthy life? As your generation ages there should be more and more of you living to be over a hundred years old. Unfortunately, it seems that your parents might have a longer average life span than your generation unless some sort of action is taken to address the poor diets and fitness habits that appear to be epidemic in our schools today. It might mean you have to sacrifice a bit now, but you just may add a few *decades* to your life and reverse the current trend.

It's time to get back to basics. It's time to realize that temptations like fast-food outlets on every corner and machines that spit out chips, soda, chocolate, and dozens of other processed foods do not offer a healthy alternative. If eating this type of food becomes a way of life for you it could easily set you on a course for future health problems you can certainly do without. The ingredients in most of the "unhealthy" foods are almost addictive. They are often manufactured in such a way that eating or drinking "just one" is sometimes not enough. That explains why eating one chocolate or one potato chip is a challenge for many people.

Once I was talking to a gentlemen who had owned a movie theater years ago, before the big theater chains took over. He told me that the admission people paid to see the movie covered his cost for renting the movie. He said where he really made a profit was on the candy, pop, and popcorn.

He even admitted that the popcorn was made in such a way that you almost *had* to buy a drink. They put extra salt in the topping to entice you to buy a soda, and the sugar in the drink makes you crave something else sweet like maybe a chocolate bar. It's a slippery slope, once you start putting excess sugar into your system. It will give you a quick burst of energy because it enters your bloodstream so fast, and you will crave more or eventually end up having a "sugar crash."

Most likely, 150 years ago, a piece of candy was something that was eaten and enjoyed a few times a year as a really special treat. It simply was not mass produced and found on every street corner and in every supermarket. It really is time to re-think what foods you should eat on a regular basis and what foods should be eaten as a very occasional treat.

Maybe it's time to eat like a caveman again. It's time for that perfect blend of carbohydrates, protein, and fat to get your body to fire on all cylinders the way it was meant to.

It seems like every week another different diet springs to life. Every day you can find someone on T.V. promoting a new weight loss product. Over my 30 year career as an endurance athlete I tried a lot of different combinations of food to see what would work best. I was constantly on the look-out for food choices that would provide the most energy and boost my endurance. I never worried about the *amount* I ate, but instead was cautious about the *quality* of the food I ate. I have never counted calories in my life, and to me it seems to be an unnecessary waste of time.

I've always believed that you should only eat the amount of food that your body needs to power you through your day. So if you are physically inactive for most of the time it makes sense that you will not be utilizing very much of what you are eating on a day to day basis. So if you over-eat, your body has little choice but to store away those extra reserves for a later date. Usually those reserves are stored as fat.

Say you decided to take up a lifestyle built around being active and fit and eating food that is more suited to fueling your body properly. As soon as you become active your body instantly springs into action to meet the new physical demands. Old muscle is broken down and replaced with new, stronger muscle. Your heart begins to strengthen as the need to pump a steady supply of blood to all those working muscles increases. You will see changes begin to take place. You have put your body on alert and it responds by getting stronger and fitter and more able to carry out these new demands.

If you plan on being in high performance mode, then it only makes sense to supply the best possible fuel for your body to work with. You will be amazed at the physical changes that will take place once you adopt a healthier, fitter lifestyle. This is the point where *what* you eat and not *how much* you eat takes on a new meaning.

For instance, when I was in triathlon training I would eat until I wasn't hungry anymore. I knew my body would tell me when it was time to fuel up and just how much I should eat. I used to call it my "appestat." So if I went out on an 80 km bike ride followed by a 10 km run it was a pretty sure bet that I would be very hungry that evening and I would eat accordingly. Sometimes I would eat huge amounts, but I made sure it was the right blend of foods. It didn't seem to matter how much I ate over the 30 years that I competed, my weight always stayed basically the same because I was burning the fuel almost as fast as I was taking it in.

Here is a perfect example of what I'm talking about. If I hadn't read this in the Globe and Mail newspaper I'm not sure I would have believed it. The article I read shortly after the Beijing Olympic Games discussed how Michael Phelps fueled himself while in intensive training. According to the article, he ate 12,000 (yes, 12,000!) calories a day in his training leading up to the Games where he went on to win 8 gold medals. Like I wrote earlier, I'm not one to count calories, but this is a staggering amount of food. To put it into perspective, the average male at that age eats about 2500 calories a day.

Obviously he needed those calories, because his body was burning them, because it sure wasn't storing any extra fat anywhere. It seems to me he would have to have been doing about 6-8 hours of intense training in an average day to burn that many calories. It seems like an impossible task, but then so does winning all those gold medals.

Eating properly is not just about losing weight. Some of you might be under the impression that you should eat as little as possible in order to remain slim and attractive. In that case, you might actually have to *gain* weight in order to reach a healthy balance. By not eating *enough* you are depriving your body of the proper nutrients it needs to maintain your overall physical health. Don't be afraid to eat lots of good wholesome food if you are balancing the food intake with fitness.

There are two main points that you should think about.

> The common denominator that makes any diet work is to include exercise along with it. The combination of eating the right foods and embracing healthy living and fitness through sports will enhance every single aspect of your life.

> Eating more than your body requires leaves it no alternative but to store it for future use. Usually that excess food is stored as fat. That means that sitting at your computer requires less fuel than if you were being physically active. Exercise and eating work best in tandem, and one without the other usually means that your body will eventually rebel.

So now, let's talk about carbohydrates, protein, and fat. It's not really all that complicated. You don't really need a dozen diet books to figure it out. You don't need to be a doctor or a scientist in order to learn how to eat healthy. If the cavemen were doing it right even before the wheel was invented, I'm sure you can as well.

Chapter Eight

* CARBOHYDRATE COMPLEXITIES *

In the past few decades, carbohydrates have been front and center in many discussions concerning diet. First they are good for you and then bad for you and then good for you again. In the rush to sell more diet books, video tapes, and super diet pills, a lot of people have been left confused and disillusioned by the latest fad that guarantees they will attain the body image they so desire. I'm sure you have lots of unanswered questions about carbohydrates. What is too much? What is too little? What do carbohydrates do? How much of it should I eat? Are some bad and are some good?

I'll tell you up front that I'm not a doctor or a scientist, but I can share with you what I've learned over the better part of 30 years of experimenting with combinations of food that would enhance my athletic ability and overall health. I truly believe there is no substitute for experience as a teaching tool, and much of what I've learned over the years will not be found in the confines of any laboratory. It took several decades to learn what combinations of foods would give me that little bit of an edge in the final 100 meters of a 10km race, push through the "wall" at the 35 km mark of a marathon, or hold things together in the last 5km of an Ironman triathlon. Through it all I learned how amazing the human body can be if treated with the respect it deserves.

I have also spent the last 40 years in the retail grocery industry, and will also give you some insight into why supermarkets are designed the way they are and the impact it has on your eating habits. This is a rare combination of information and thoughts on two entirely different aspects of the world of nutrition, and hopefully it will help you find your way as you embark on your journey toward a healthier and fitter way of life.

It's important to remember that carbohydrates come in two basic categories. They can be either *simple* or *complex* carbohydrates. I can't stress enough how important it is that you understand the difference between the two and learn how to identify what carbohydrates belong in what group. Over the years, one of the most important things I've learned concerning nutrition is that *complex* carbohydrates are the foundation of a sound and healthy diet. It's the complex carbohydrates that are the fuel for the fire that burns fat and converts it into energy. So it only makes sense that the majority of the carbohydrates you eat should be complex.

It speaks volumes for the value of complex carbohydrates when you consider that most Asian cultures have a diet high in complex carbohydrates and have few problems with weight and in fact often live to be well over 100 years old and still remain physically and mentally sharp. The cornerstones of their excellent diet is rice, vegetables, fruit, and fish.

There are many different schools of thought on what percentage of food intake should be carbohydrate. One popular combination is 40% carbohydrates, 30% protein, and 30% fat. There was also a diet craze a few years back that was mostly protein and a minimum of carbohydrates. I try not to write about something I have never experienced for myself, so despite my misgivings I tried that high protein diet in order to gauge the results for myself and it was a disaster. Within a matter of days my energy levels took a dive. Especially because I was training on a regular basis. From my experience, the right balance of complex carbohydrates will always be King in the world of healthy nutrition, and I would never suggest to anyone that eating more protein than carbohydrates is a good idea. If you are physically active and deprive your body of carbohydrates you will come to a full stop very quickly.

I'm going to give you a little test so you can see where you are as far as understanding the difference between simple and complex carbohydrates. How many complex carbohydrates can you find in this set of foods?

Muffin	Bagel	Donut	Orange
Fruit Juice	Chocolate Bar	Pickle	Slice of Cake
Whole Wheat Bread	Timbit	Carrot	Pita Bread
Your Mom's Apple Pie	Ice Cream	Cookie	Baked Potato
Granola Bar	Energy Gel	Apple	Honey
Can of Pop (Soda)	Licorice		

Well, how did you make out? It's really important to make the distinction between simple and complex when it comes to your carbohydrate choices, because that is where the secret to increased energy, weight loss, and endurance will be found.

There are five complex carbohydrates on the above list. The five healthiest choices on that list are whole wheat bread, bagel, potato, pita bread, and a carrot. The rest are all simple carbohydrates. I'm sure there is food on that list that you have eaten that has given you an instant burst of energy, followed by a sugar crash that left you feeling tired and listless. Your choice might have been a can of pop and a chocolate bar, for instance. As good as they might taste, they have a way of making you feel crappy shortly after you eat them. That in itself should show the impact a poor nutrition source can have on your body's ability to perform at optimum levels.

All simple carbohydrates are not created equal, and I'm not saying they are *all* poor choices. Fruit, for example, should definitely be part of your daily diet, but not extreme amounts. The reason they are considered a simple carbohydrate is because of their sugar content, but they still should be part of your diet because of the vitamins and fiber they provide. If your goal is to have 6 or 8 servings of fruit or vegetables on average per day then just make a point of making the greater percentage of the servings vegetables.

Remember that a large salad is not considered *one* serving. If it's a large salad it's probably more like 4 servings. So if you have just one large salad per day, two serving of vegetables with your meals and two fruit choices(like maybe a banana with breakfast or in a smoothie and an apple for a snack between meals), then you have had your 8 servings of fruit and vegetables for the day.

If you can remember this comparison it will help you understand the difference between simple and complex carbohydrates. If you were to drink a big glass of pure apple juice it would be assimilated into your bloodstream almost immediately, mostly because it's loaded with natural sugar. It's easily broken down by your body and assimilated. Well, as a matter of fact, it's "simple."

On the other hand, a salad full of tomatoes, celery, lettuce, cucumbers, green onions, or any other fresh vegetables you might happen to include present more of a challenge for your body to break down. The work effort required is more "complex" and as a result the carbohydrates from your salad are absorbed by your body over a longer period of time. In a nutshell, that's why you get a quick surge of energy from a chocolate bar, a pop, or anything else loaded with sugar. It goes almost straight into your bloodstream. It actually causes an insulin imbalance and that's why often a sugar crash or energy loss is the end result.

Complex carbohydrates will provide fuel that will sustain you over a longer period of time. That's why athletes load up on pasta, salads, rice, and whole wheat bread the day before the big event. They realize the complex carbohydrates in these foods will help provide energy over a longer period of time and enhance their strength and endurance as a result.

Personally I found that 50% carbohydrates, 25% protein, and 25% fat was the perfect balance for my active lifestyle. Of that

50% carbohydrates, at least 40% should be complex and 10% can be simple like fruit, fruit juice, gels, and sports drinks. Remember that fruit juice and sports drinks have quite a lot of sugar so be careful not to over-do it. Water will always be King when it comes to hydrating your body.

The whole grain carbohydrates are best. Whole wheat bread, buns, bagels, pasta, oatmeal, and brown rice are some excellent choices. Potatoes are also an excellent choice when balanced with protein. They were the cornerstone of my diet when I was training the hardest. I also made a point of eating a big salad at least five or six times a week.

The process of eating and fueling your body is not all that complicated. You fuel your body, you burn that fuel, and you replace it. Since the beginning of time this process has never changed. What has changed is how we as a society have lost sight of the basic fundamentals of what *good* food truly is.

I can't stress how important it is that you begin to look at pop, chocolate, donuts, cake, and the other junk food filled with sugar, salt, and fat as treats to be enjoyed very, very rarely and not a staple part of your diet. This is absolutely critical, and is a thought process you should adopt as soon as possible.

Making this one conscious decision about the way you fuel your body has the power to change your life forever.

Believe me, that's not an exaggeration.

Chapter Nine

PROTEIN POWER

There's no doubt that protein is essential to maintaining your muscle tissue, organs, bones, and immune system. This is true on an everyday basis, but when you are physically active and working out, it's even more essential to include quality protein in your diet. As you stress your muscles, the old tissue breaks down and is replaced with new tissue. That's the reason why you should alternate workout days with rest days if you are on a weight lifting program. By giving the muscles you just stressed a rest day you are allowing your body time to begin the rebuilding process. That's why most body-builders will work their upper body one day and their lower body the next.

Personally, when I incorporated weight training into my triathlon training program I did a full body workout each session and took every other day off. I lifted weights three days per week and took the weekends off. I also made a point of eating a little extra protein when I was lifting weights. Even if you don't do weight training, it's important to always have adequate protein in your diet, but when you are putting extra stress on your muscles, it's even more important as your body works overtime to build newer stronger muscle. Protein shakes with protein powder, soy milk, frozen banana, and a raw egg were one of my favorite protein treats.

It's also protein that your body will use to manufacture hemoglobin. That's the part of your red blood cells that makes sure oxygen gets to where it is needed in your body, and that's pretty well everywhere. Some proteins help build your heart muscle and even when you're not moving around, protein is always working away protecting you from disease.

The protein you eat is broken down into units called amino acids. Of all the amino acids found in protein, there are around 22 that are most important to your health. Fortunately our bodies can make 13 of them with little effort, but the other nine require you to eat food rich in protein. Those are what are called "essential amino acids" because it's important to get them from the food you eat.

Carbohydrates, protein, and fat complement each other and ensure you get the nutrition you need. Peanuts on their own might not supply all the essential amino acids you need, but if you spread peanut butter on whole-grain bread, you will have a much better chance of meeting your needs. If you maintain well-balanced meals throughout the day your body will be able to sort out all the amino acids it needs to do its work.

There are numerous foods that contain protein, but some of the best sources are beef, poultry, fish, nuts, eggs, and most dairy products. Consider using skim milk if you do use milk on a regular basis. If the protein is from an animal source like milk or beef, it's called *complete*. That's because it contains the nine essential amino acids that you are missing.

The same can't be said for vegetable protein and it's called *incomplete* because it's usually missing at least one of the essential amino acids. That's why it's important for vegetarians to eat a wide variety of vegetables that are rich in proteins. That way there is a better chance of getting all the essential amino acids necessary to rebuild their body.

There are many different equations out there that will suggest how many grams of protein you need according to your size and age etc., but really, it doesn't have to be that complicated. There are many different opinions on how to break down the percentages of carbohydrates, proteins, and fats you should eat on a given day. Personally after years of trial and error I found that trying to make my food intake about 25-30% protein was about right. You don't have to be weighing, counting and balancing everything you eat in order to judge the perfect proportions. In time you will get a feel for just the right amount of protein you should be eating.

For instance if you had a serving of pasta, a piece of chicken about half the size of the pasta serving would be about the right amount of protein to balance that meal. If you want a visual guideline to help you balance the protein in your meals, imagine having two handfuls of a carbohydrate like rice or potatoes, or pasta, and one handful of protein. It might be fish, chicken or lean beef for example. If you feel you need more protein because you have done some swimming, biking or weight-lifting that day, you can always make yourself a protein shake. Just experiment with some of the ingredients I mentioned until you find a combination that you enjoy. I always used to prefer cutting up ripe bananas and freezing them. They turn your smoothie into a healthy milkshake. Both peanut butter and almond butter are rich in quality protein and can boost your protein intake on any given day if you feel you have not had enough. However, be sure it's pure peanuts with nothing added. It's a little more expensive than the peanut butter with additives, but is much better for you. you can always tell if it's the real thing because the oil will rise to the top of natural peanut butter and you will have to stir it in. If you look at the ingredients list, all it should say is "peanuts" and nothing else.

Peanut or almond butter would also be great choices for vegetarians as well who are in search of quality, meat-free protein. Again, imagine spreading the nut butter on a slice of whole wheat bread. There is your perfect 50% carbohydrate 25% protein balance. Of course if you are allergic to nuts you might have to look for an alternative spreads to put on your whole wheat bread. Possibly you could look into the use of hemp seed butter. It is actually even a better source of fat and protein than peanut butter, and although very expensive is an alternative you might consider.

You might also try using cottage cheese as a topping for your salads. This is a far healthier choice than the salad dressings loaded with sugar and poor quality fats. My choice of cottage cheese was the 1% milk fat variety. Plain yogurt is another dairy product high in protein and mixed with a fresh fruit of your choice can be a healthy snack. There are many yogurt choices out there that have far too much sugar in them, and it's far better to buy the plain variety and add your own fruit.

Keep in mind that over-eating proteins does not necessarily make you grow stronger at a faster pace. Your body will use what it needs and the rest will be turned into fat, so try to avoid eating more than you actually need in the hopes that it will get you where you want to go even faster. Your body simply does not work that way, and will follow the master plan that was set down eons ago. Like a maestro leading the orchestra, Mother Nature will skillfully combine the essential high quality nutrients you eat and create the beautiful music that results when your body is operating at its highest level.

Chapter Ten

* FABULOUS FAT *

Fat is not necessarily your enemy, and is just as essential as carbohydrates and protein to your health and well-being.

The key is to ensure that the fats you eat are of the highest quality and not the dangerous and unhealthy fats that are found in so many food products on the market today.

It would be easy to get bogged-down discussing good and bad cholesterol, and the whole range of ills caused by unhealthy fats. I will leave that to the scientists, doctors, and other experts and concentrate on the food choices that contain the quality fats that were instrumental in keeping me fit and healthy over my 30 year career as an endurance athlete and some of the food choices I never touched if I was after optimum results.

I will attempt to list some of the better food choices for you when it comes to providing quality fat that will work in tandem with clean burning complex carbohydrates and provide your body with the power, endurance, and energy you need to fuel your new-found high performance lifestyle.

Much like protein, it's not necessary to exactly measure the amount of fat you are eating every day. Keep in mind that fat will be present in many of the foods that are high in carbohydrates and protein. Some excellent examples are eggs, peanut butter, and almond butter. All three food items are high in quality protein as well as quality fat.

The key when it comes to fats is to make healthy food choices on a daily basis. It doesn't take an expert to figure out that peanut butter on whole wheat bread is better for you than a bag of potato chips. One contains fat that will help fuel your body and the other has fat that will help clog your arteries.

A good ratio of fat in your diet is about 25-30%. It will fluctuate depending on the amounts and quality of carbohydrates and protein you are eating. It's important to note that attention should be given to the *quality* of the fat you eat and not so much the *quantity*.

If you were to take a meal of potatoes, chicken, a serving of vegetables, and a salad, here is how you might add in the fat. First of all, there is fat in the chicken. You could use a little butter on the potatoes and that is also fat. When I was being really strict with what I ate I would put 1% cottage cheese on my baked potatoes instead of butter and sour cream. Cottage cheese also contains a good quality fat. Years ago my choice of dressing for my salads became red wine vinegar and EVOO. Put that on your salad instead of one of those dressings full of poor fats and sugar.

I will spell that out for you. Extra Virgin Olive Oil (EVOO). So ask your parents to buy you some EVOO unless of course they already have it in the cupboard.

Remember that name because it's an amazing source of healthy fat. EVOO far surpasses canola and vegetable oils when it comes to a fat that will complement the high quality carbohydrates and protein you eat. There was a period in the mid 1900's when the Greeks had the highest life expectancy in the world and it was attributed to their diet that was very high in nuts and olive oil. Once they started to include processed foods into their diet and the saturated fats that came along with it, they started to develop more heart related disease and began to die at at an earlier age.

It was years later when I began to do research on *coconut oil*. It's also a very good fat and has some qualities that make it one of the more unique and beneficial oils in the world.

In a nutshell, coconut oil is comprised of fatty acids called "medium chain triglycerides". In fact, in all of nature, coconut oil has one of the highest concentrations of these MCTs. On the other hand, vegetable oil is primarily made up of "long chain fatty acids" (LCTs).

These LCTs tend to produce fat in your body, but MTCs increase your body's metabolism and create energy, and as a result, decrease your body fat.

I put it into practice and began using coconut oil while I was in full triathlon training. I started out with one tablespoon a day and over time increased my intake to four tablespoons per day. I used it in my smoothies, pasta sauce, pasta, rice, and used it in any recipe that called for butter or margarine. In three or four weeks I started to notice an increase in energy, and even though I wasn't trying to, I actually lost weight for the first time in years. I didn't think I had any excess weight to lose, but somehow coconut oil managed to find it and eliminate it. For the most part my weight never varied much for over 30 years. So I knew with a certainty that it was the coconut oil that had caused the weight loss.

The key is to be active while you are using coconut oil. It seems to be a combination of being active while using coconut oil that increase metabolism resulting in the weight loss. In other words, coconut oil is a fat that seems to burn fat.

You can buy very expensive organic "virgin" coconut oil that retains the coconut flavor, or you can purchase the less expensive brands that work just as well but don't have as strong a coconut scent and taste.

There are also certain fish that are very high in fat content. Salmon is an excellent choice for unsaturated fat and is full of Omega-3 fatty acids. These acids are excellent for the health of your heart and even have beneficial effects in certain depressive disorders.

Our earliest ancestors to ever walk the earth were well aware of the importance of fat in their diet. Evidence that seems to verify that was uncovered at various archaeological sites. At many of the sites it was not unusual to find animal bones that had been split open. It's believed that the caveman was using the marrow inside as a source of fat. It's also believed that in some cases they left the meat of the animals and hunted them strictly for their bones.

They hunted the woolly mammoth, sloth, bears, bison, and wild pigs, as most of these animals came with a fairly thick layer of subcutaneous fat. Scientists also believe that if they follow the patterns of today's African hunter-gatherers, the caveman most likely preferred the organs, brains, tongue and feet of their prey because of the fat content.

The Eskimo has long known the importance of fat and the seal and the whale became important parts of their diet. They also reasoned that the best time to hunt elk was after they had a chance to feed on the grasses of the tundra at certain times of the year. Otherwise they would be too lean, and have no fat. The Eskimo realized that if all they ate was lean meat, they would leave themselves open to a variety of sicknesses.

So don't hesitate to include fat in your diet. Fat is just as important as protein and carbohydrates are to your health and well-being. The first humans to ever walk the earth realized that and nothing has changed. It's just important now as it was then.

The key is to make sure that the fats you choose are high quality and not the saturated fats that are found in most of today's processed and fast foods.

Chapter Eleven

* SPICE IT UP *

Often our fridges and cupboards are full of those tricky treats that we *add* to our meals in order to kick them up a notch.

These are called condiments, and all of them are not created equal. By themselves, they might not seem like a big deal, but if you are continually covering your food with ketchup, sauces, relishes, processed cheese, salt, salad dressings, and dozens of other not so healthy toppings out there, they will soon add up and stall your forward progress to higher standard of nutrition. They also tend to mask the true flavor of the food you are eating.

After a while you will get really good at picking out the best condiments to add to your diet. You will find alternatives you never knew existed and perhaps for the first time begin to taste the real flavor of some foods.

For example, try using red wine vinegar (or even lemon juice) and olive oil as a dressing for your salad instead of one of those dressings loaded with sugar and fat. Even the ones that say "diet" can be very deceiving. When I started using that simple combination of olive oil and vinegar, I really started to enjoy the flavor of the vegetables in the salad a lot more.

I have this vision of a caveman pulling a root out of the ground and pouring ketchup on it. It boggles the mind, yet people do it all the time whenever they see a French fry.

Always look for the best alternative when you are looking for the healthiest way to eat. Maybe use salsa instead of ketchup. Quality oil instead of sugary dressings. Olive oil instead of vegetable oil. Skim milk instead of whole milk. Sea salt instead of iodized salt. Fresh fruit before frozen fruit, and frozen fruit before canned fruit. Fresh vegetables before frozen vegetables and frozen vegetables before canned vegetables. (but whatever you do, eat your vegetables, even though you still might not get dessert if your mom gets her hands on this book). Hard cheeses instead of processed cheese. For instance Parmesan is the best choice for cheese as a topping. It's great on pasta and you can always put it on your salads if you want a bit of a different flavor. Cheddar cheese is a good choice, but limit the amount you eat as there is quite a lot of fat in it.

When it comes to spices my two favorites are pepper and cinnamon (not cinnamon *sugar*, just cinnamon). They add tons of flavor to so many dishes and are a way better choice than putting salt and sugar on everything. Try cinnamon on your oatmeal, on your whole wheat pancakes, and in your smoothie.

Add fruit to your meals in places you have maybe never tried. When you make your smoothie, throw in some fresh or frozen strawberries or blueberries. Try putting blueberries in your whole wheat pancakes and topping with 100% apple sauce and cinnamon instead of syrup.

Put fruit in your vegetable salad. For instance you might try sliced fresh peaches when they are in season. Sliced apples and grapes also go great with vegetables and give your salad a new, healthy flavor. You might be used to vegetables and fruits being separated in cooking and in recipes, but experiment and try combining them for a new taste experience.

Instead of adding sugar to your oatmeal, try adding a handful of raisins, a tablespoon of coconut oil, a sprinkle of cinnamon and topping with a little skim milk.

Use your imagination and you will find there are many healthy ways to make everyday food taste great and at the same time be eating smart.

Chapter Twelve

* LABEL ME *

It would be very wise to get used to turning food products over and reading the label. By law, manufacturers must record everything that is in the product. Normally the percentage of each additive determines its order on the list. The more of an additive the food has, the higher it is on the list. In other words if the first few things you see on a label are salt, sugar, and three names you, your teacher, your mother, and I can't pronounce, then most likely it's not a great choice for you.

If it says hydrogenated oil, it's not a great choice. If it says saturated fat, it's not a great choice. Potato chips will usually have potatoes, some kind of fat, and salt at the top of the list. Ketchup will have syrup or some other bizarre sweetener at the top of the list. In almost all of today's foods you will find added fat, salt, and sugar of one kind or another.

Here is a quiz for you. I will give you the ingredients for a food item available in the frozen food section of your local supermarket and see if you know what it is...

> Enriched flour, water, vegetable oil shortening, hydrogenated vegetable soybean and cottonseed oil, sorbitan tristerate color, salt, dough conditioner, wheat flour l-cystene hydrochlorde-alpha amlase, cream of tartar, sodium propanate, ground beef, bread crumbs, flour, durham flour leavening, sodium bicarbonate, sodium acid pyrophosphate, dried yeast, corn starch, dehydrated onions, salt yeast extract, corn syrup, caramel, brown sugar, tavarid concentrate, onion powder and liquid egg white.

Well, how did you do?

If you guessed sausage roll, you're the winner. It's hard to imagine so many mystery ingredients can be packed into something so small. Worse yet, one serving has 28 g of mostly poor quality saturated and trans fats and 600 mg of sodium. Mmmmm.

Now, let's look at the ingredients list for oatmeal:
　　Oats.

Well, that's the list of ingredients for oatmeal and can there be any question why it might be the healthier of these two food choices?

Here is a list of ingredients that are similar to about 99% of the peanut butter you will find on supermarket shelves.

> Peanuts, Maltodextrin, Icing Sugar, Soybean Oil, Salt, Hydrogenated Vegetable Oil, Monoglyceride.

Most of the additives in peanut butter are in there to give it that smooth, creamy texture, but really what's happened is that a good source of protein and fat has been turned into something far different and not nearly as healthy.

Here are the ingredients for "Natural" peanut butter.

> Peanuts.

... Hmmm.

If you look closely, you may find some of the natural variety on your next trip to the supermarket. When you get natural peanut butter home and open it, you will most likely find that the oil has naturally settled on top of the peanut butter. You will have to stir it back in. It can be a bit messy, but it's well worth the inconvenience. Once it's back to being smooth again, just keep it in the refrigerator and you will not have to stir it again.

When you are looking for something to spice up your meals or are unsure if something is a healthy or unhealthy choice, just turn it over and read the label. If there are a lot of names on that label you don't understand, then most likely it is full of preservatives, unhealthy fats and many other additives that you will be putting into your system if you choose to eat them. Pay special attention to *trans fats, saturated fats,* and *hydrogenated fats* appearing on the label. Also look out for syrups, sugars, and other sweeteners.

Sure, most processed foods seem okay because they taste good and you don't seem to have any ill effects, but over time, making poor nutrition choices will have a telling effect on your long term health and longevity. It's a sad fact that what makes food appear to taste good to us is fat, salt, and sugar. If you take those away, many people find food bland. That's mostly because you've acquired a taste for that sugar and fat. In effect, you may have become addicted to it, and though it may take a while to get used to healthy eating, it opens up a whole new world of flavor and health for you.

In the history of the world, the years ahead of you may well be the most incredible in all of creation. Expect to see huge advances in medicine in your lifetime. Most likely you will witness the elimination of cancer and other illnesses that have plagued humanity for centuries. Advances that should make living up to 100 years old, and longer, quite common. You could well see colonies on the moon and cars that drive themselves. Who knows, you could even be taking a holiday to Mars in your retirement years.

However, as things stand now, your generation might have a life expectancy that's shorter than your parents'. That should never happen, but it very well might because of the nature of the times you have been born into.

Something as easy to change as the way you nourish and care for your body could well make the difference between living to be 60 or 100 years old or more. What amazing wonders you will get to see as you pass through adulthood and into your senior years if you are still healthy and fit and around to enjoy all the world has to offer as the year 2100 gets nearer.

Being aware of everything you are giving your body to work with in the way of nourishment is a great start to living strong and healthy for many, many years. Take control of your destiny by questioning, experimenting and learning all there is to know about the world of food.

Everything you do and everything you are focuses around nutrition. There is simply no escaping it. You will always have to eat, so why not find the best way?

Chapter Thirteen

* MILES OF AISLES *

I'm nearing the end of four decades in the retail grocery industry. In that time I've seen first hand or have been involved in pretty much every aspect of the day to day operations of a grocery supermarket.

I've witnessed many changes in the inner workings of food stores in relation to the consumer and the way people in general have changed their eating habits and the many new products they have been inundated with over the years.

There is an ebb and flow to the grocery industry that hinges on what the consumer demands, the latest fads in nutrition, and of course from the point of view of any company, making a profit.

Some of the changes I've witnessed have been good ones. For

instance, I remember when yogurt was something hardly anyone ever ate and it had very little room on the shelf. At most, maybe a few feet. Now stores have *huge* sections in the dairy department just for yogurt. Instead of selling a few containers a day, stores now sell yogurt of every type and description by the hundreds every single week.

Supermarkets are always on the lookout for the latest fad diets that will most likely result in the consumer looking for specific food items. Whether the diet is good for you or not isn't their concern. Their concern is meeting the demand and making a profit. A good example is the diet touting high protein and almost zero carbohydrates that swept across North America several years ago. Within months we had these high protein, low carbohydrate products all over the store. It was probably less than a year later that people woke up and realized it was a really poor concept for a diet. Once the demand was gone, the products disappeared from the shelves and were no longer sold in the store.

I worked in the produce department for many years and was

there when it evolved to become one of the most important departments in any grocery store. I saw many new items the day they arrived in the stores for the first time. Take the kiwi fruit, for example. None of us knew what those little brown things were the first time they arrived with our produce order. We would put one case out on display and then throw it out when it turned bad because nobody bought them. Customers didn't know what they were, either. Once people gave them a try and realized they were very flavorful and a great source of potassium and other nutrients as well, they became very popular and still are to this day.

Next came all the new varieties of apples from around the world. I remember the first time we ever sold a "Granny Smith" apple. Then came Gala, Jonagold, Fuji, and a host of new varieties that were new to us and the entire country for that matter.

You know those bagged salads you see in the produce department? When they first came out there were a few varieties that had a couple of feet of shelf space. Most of us in the business thought they would never last. Who on earth would buy an expensive bag of ready made salad when they could make their own for half the price? Well, it turns out the timing was just perfect to introduce the salad in a bag as people began to count more and more on making meals that were quick and easy. Now some stores have shelves 20 feet (6 meters) long and 5 shelves high full of those salads and they can never keep them full.

To me that was a positive and healthy change that inspired more people to eat salads who otherwise might not have bothered.

The next biggest positive change was the introduction of *organic* produce to the shopping public. Food grown without pesticides, herbicides, or any other chemicals are in demand by consumers who want the healthiest choices possible when it comes to their nutrition.

Unfortunately, there is often not a sufficient supply of organic produce, as it takes more effort to grow, and the cost to the consumer can be quite high, so for now, many average families simply can't afford it. I, for one, can envision the day in the near future when more and more back yard gardens will begin to take over lawns and flower beds as people come to the realization that going back to the land is not such a bad idea.

Those are some of the more positive changes I've seen in the retail food industry, but there have been many that are not so positive and are not so great for you, the young adult who was born into a world of fast food and convenience and downright *bad* eating habits by the majority of the population of North America.

It's very true that we are all a product of our environment.

Say, for example, you were born 100 years ago into a family that lived on a farm. The food you would eat was food that was for the most part nurtured and grown on the family farm. Your vegetables came from the garden and your meat, eggs and milk came from the farm animals. You and your mother might even go out and pick wild berries for the pie she would make for

Sunday dinner. Maybe once a month the family would ride into town and buy the staple items they needed at the general store and maybe then, you would even get a bit of candy for a treat.

Is it any wonder that farm boys grew big and strong, and farm girls had beautiful hair and skin and were healthy and gorgeous? There were no fast food outlets, no soft drinks, potato chips, chocolate, processed foods or numerous other unhealthy food choices to tempt them.

The one word to describe the way they lived and the body image they projected might be *wholesome.*

Now look at the world you were born into.

From the moment you could walk you were pushing one of those little carts through the grocery aisles when your parents did the weekly shopping. As a people, we have gone from living off the land to living off the aisles and aisles of grocery shelves. Those grocery aisles were your introduction to the world of food as it exists today.

How could it possibly *not* influence the way your nutrition habits were formed as you grew up?

This is an example of what you will most likely see when you walk down the aisles of any modern day supermarket.

You will see 50-80 feet (15.24-24.38 meters) of sugar-laden soft drinks that are on shelves that will be almost 2 feet deep and about 4 rows high, but there will only be about 12 or so feet (3.65 meters) of bottled water and sports drinks.

You will see 60-80 feet (18.28-24.38 meters) of potato chips also 4 or 5 rows high, but only a very few are not loaded with salt and fat.

You will see almost 20 feet (6.09 meters) of ice cream products in most stores, but about 12 feet (3.65 meters) of frozen vegetables.

You will see 16-20 feet (4.87-6.09 meters) of candies and

chocolate bars, about 9 feet (2.74 meters) of that microwave popcorn that's loaded with very poor quality fat and salt, and maybe one lonely shelf of real popcorn kernels that are a healthy snack and only have one ingredient on the package: Corn.

Then you will turn down the cereal aisle and look toward the far end about 70 feet (21.33) away at box after box of sugar bombs that make kids bounce off the walls and ceiling as the sugar goes directly into their bloodstream. As a little kid this might have been one of your favorite aisles in the whole store. Well, next to the candy and ice cream aisles, anyway.

When I was attempting to eat the healthiest possible diet to go along with my training, there were only about 4 different cereals in that entire aisle that I would eat.

Puffed wheat, puffed rice, shredded wheat, and oatmeal.

In order these are the ingredients in those 4 cereals: wheat, rice, wheat, and oats.   Period.

When you look at the ingredients list on pretty well every box of cereal in that aisle, one of the first thing you will see is salt and sugar on that list. When I wanted the very best, I would never buy it if it had additives of any kind.

The four cereals I just listed are all whole grains and have nothing added. It was up to me to add what *I* thought best. So, for example, I would sometimes put raisins, banana, or apple in my oatmeal. I would sprinkle it with cinnamon and mix in a tablespoon of coconut oil while it cooked and top it off with some skim milk.

So that was *my* list of additives. Fruit, cinnamon, organic virgin coconut oil, and skim milk. If you take control of what you are eating you will be aware of everything you are feeding your body, and you will eliminate the mystery ingredients that may be detrimental to your health. Instead of factory engineered chemical additives, my bowl of cereal contained excellent quality complex carbohydrates in the oatmeal, desirable simple carbohydrates in the fruit, protein in the milk, and an excellent source of fat in the coconut oil and also in the oatmeal itself. Add a few pieces of lightly buttered whole wheat toast and a small glass of pure orange juice and you have a well-balanced, nutritional breakfast fit for a King.

The last thing you will see when you check out with your groceries in most grocery stores is most likely going to be coolers full of pop and more shelves of chocolate bars and candies. Those are called "impulse" sales and are there to temp you one last time. They are there to trigger that sweet tooth and sugar craving that always seems to be present in most people. The reason it's there is because like millions of others, you have become addicted to sugar. You just don't realize it.

This is the world of food you have been born into. This is what has most likely shaped the nutrition habits you have right now.

You have become a product of your environment.

Yes, a lot of the blame should be placed on big business who want to make a profit at the expense of your health and yet at the same time don't feel responsible for the way you choose to eat. It's the rationale of supply and demand and free enterprise. As long as people crave it and will buy it, the stores will stock it and sell it. If all of a sudden the consumer bought half as much ice cream and twice as many frozen vegetables, then at corporate headquarters somewhere a computer would spit out the new trend and soon the shelf space that was allocated would be reconfigured and you would see twice as many vegetables than ice cream instead of the other way around.

Supply and demand. If people demand it, stores will supply it.

When you go into a supermarket they are designed to keep traffic flowing through every aisle, yet if you are intent on adopting a healthier way of eating, 90% of your shopping should actually be done along the side walls and back wall of any store. When you enter the supermarket, the produce department will most likely be on wall to your left or right. The other wall will most likely be the bakery and deli and the back wall will be the dairy and meat department.

If you are intent on eating healthy you would be wise to do the majority of your shopping along those three walls. Sure you might venture into the center aisles for a few specific healthy foods and non food items you might need. Possibly you will look for spices, pasta or rice. You will also find the healthy cereals I mentioned, raisins, natural peanut butter, olive oil, frozen vegetables or perhaps canned fish and a few other healthy food choices that will enhance your diet.

The fact is, the more control you have over what you eat and the more discerning you are, the less time you are going to spend in those miles of aisles. You will be in and out to get the specific healthy products you want and leave behind the thousands of other poor nutrition choices that are bombarding consumers every time they turn around.

It's unfortunate, but I truly believe that you as a young adult might be under the impression that because adults sell certain things, that it automatically means that it's okay and won't be a bad choice for you.

The truth is, because our society is based on free enterprise and anyone can sell pretty well anything they want, the onus is on the consumer to know what's good for them or not good for them. The retailer will do anything he can to entice you to buy his product with little regard for how it will impact your health or your life. That's simply the way of the world we live in.

Stores sell cigarettes, yet they kill thousands of people every year. Everyone knows it, and yet they are still sold to the general public. Stores sell alcohol, and yet every year hundreds die in North America because of impaired driving.

There is a message here that is blaring out to you in big, bold letters. It's the same message I gave you at the beginning of this book.

Take control and responsibility for your life now!

You have the power within you to decide what's best for *you* and to not be seduced by T.V. ads or merchandising practices of retail businesses who for the most part are more concerned about profit than your health and well-being. Just because something is there staring you in the face or it is somehow glamorized, does not make it a good choice and does not make it right.

That goes for poor food choices, alcohol, cigarettes, and anything else that can have an enormous negative impact on the way you live your life.

You only have so much time in this world, and how you live it is in your hands.

Remember that often ill health takes years to develop. Heart problems often seem to be caused by years and sometimes decades of poor living habits. So you may think it's not so bad if you have 3 soft drinks a day and fast food 5 times a week, because at the time it tastes great. So what if you get out of breath easy and you seem to be gaining more weight every month?

The truth is, whatever decisions you make concerning your

nutrition right now will go a long way toward determining the quality of the rest of your life and how and when you depart this world.

I'll leave you with this story.

About 15 years ago I wanted to earn extra money to help pay my expenses when I went to races etc. I found a part-time job working with this man who ran his own business working on the exteriors of new houses. I would work with him on my days off from my full-time job.

At noon everyday we would stop and take an hour for lunch. My boss would open up his lunch bucket full of these big sandwiches made up of cheese and processed meat in big white buns, maybe a can of pop, a few donuts, a big piece of chocolate cake or a piece of pie.

Almost always I would take a tuna sandwich on brown bread, a bottle of water, and an apple or banana out of my lunch bag. He always got a laugh out of that.

Usually after I finished a full day's work with him, I would head home and go for a 15 km run or maybe a 50km bike training ride because I had some big races coming up later that year. I had no problem doing that while working 7 days a week at the time.

My boss would go home and sit around until supper time and not do much else until it was time to come back to work the next day.

It was obvious that he was overweight and one day when we were having lunch and talking, I asked him if it ever worried about how his eating habits might effect his future health. I'll never forget what he said to me.

He said, "I would rather eat everything I want everyday and enjoy it. If I eat food I don't really enjoy I might live 5 years longer but not enjoy eating."

At the time he was nearing 60 and was about ready to quit the working life and retire. I thought for a long time about what he had said that day and no matter which way I looked at it, it just didn't make sense to me. I mean, he had a wife and grown kids. Wouldn't it make more sense to live a longer, healthier life, and be able to spend that much more time with them? Especially if all it would take was a healthier way of eating and a some fitness added to his lifestyle.

Right or wrong, it is up to you to make that same choice for yourself. You can abuse your body all you want and live (or die) with the results, or you can embrace a life of healthy nutrition and fitness and give yourself the best possible chance to live a long, healthy, productive life far into your senior years. Of course there are no guarantees, but at least you are doing the best you can.

Oh, and my boss? Shortly after he retired he had a heart attack and died. He was 61 years old.

When I heard the news I was very sad, because he was a good person, but I consoled myself with the knowledge that he had made his decision. It just seemed like such a shame to me because just by modifying his diet a bit and staying physically active throughout his life he could have easily lived another 20 or 25 healthy years. They would have been very special years he could have spent enjoying retirement and extra time with family and friends.

As for myself, I still have my oatmeal about 3 times a week and have a salad at least 5 days a week, and still enjoy my tuna sandwiches on whole wheat bread. I'm 59 and have my sights set on running competitively well into my 70's. If it's not meant to be for some reason that's fine, but it certainly won't be because I lost sight of how important diet and fitness are in the big scheme of things.

Simply changing some lifestyle patterns that have been imprinted in your brain because of the world you have been born into can pay *huge* dividends in later years and give you the best possible chance to live a long, healthy, and productive life.

Chapter Fourteen

On the last Sunday of August 2008, the Ironman Canada triathlon took place in Penticton, B.C.

The Ironman Triathlon consists of a 3.8 km swim, 180 km bike, and a full marathon of 42.2 km. All three disciplines must be completed in 17 hours in order to be considered an official finisher.

Of the 2300 entries who began the swim when the cannon went off to begin the race that Sunday morning in August there were 7 men entered in the 70-74 age group. There was also a woman in the 75-79 age-group. There were entries from 18 to 78, and every age in between. In any given summer there are kids from 4 years old to teens who also compete in shorter distance triathlons all over the world. So as you can see, triathlon is indeed a sport for everyone and is the reason it has become one of the fastest growing sports in the world.

So if you need a sport that would be a good starting place for you to get physically fit and have fun at the same time, triathlon might be the perfect choice for you.

Here are some of the reasons I think it's a sport you might consider.

> It's a sport for all ages and all levels of athletic ability.

> You can progress at your own speed.

> It doesn't matter if you are athletic and strong or new to sports and just trying to get into better shape.

> You don't have to make a team in order to be able to take part.

> There is no coach you have to impress.

> It's an opportunity to learn some new skills. For instance, if

you can't swim, you can take lessons and learn how. Being able to swim is a great skill because over the years you will most likely be around water many times and knowing how to swim could save your life or the life of someone else one day.

➢ There are three different sports to learn about and train for. That way you never have to do the same thing over and over again. One day you might swim and the next you might bike or maybe one day you will run and then bike.

➢ You can take the sport as far as you want. You can take part just to have fun and stay fit or you can go all the way to the Olympics one day. Simon Whitfield started out having fun and being fit and since then has been in the Olympics 3 times and has won a gold and silver medal.

➢ It's not a really expensive sport. To start with all you need is a bike and helmet, a swim suit and swim goggles, and a pair of running shoes, a t-shirt or singlet, and shorts, and you are ready to go! If you really, really get to like the sport, there is plenty of time to think about buying more expensive equipment one day.

Triathlon, along with good nutrition, will help you get in the best shape of your life, and you will meet some very cool people who are interested in being fit just like you are. Of course, like most sports, there will be rules and regulations you will have to learn and be aware of that are essential to safety and fair play.

Another thing that makes triathlon a great sport is that you will be competing within your age group. That is usually determined by your age on December 31st of the year of competition.

Kids as young as 4 or 5 can enter certain races, but normally the youngest age group will be 6 and 7 year olds. They might swim 50 meters, bike 1.5 kilometers, and finish with a 500 meter run.

The next two age groups are 8 and 9 year olds and 10 and 11 year olds. They might swim 100 meters, bike 5 kilometers, and run 1 kilometer. The emphasis is on fun. At this age, some kids get competitive, but it doesn't mean you have to. You just go at whatever speed suits you.

If you are 12 or 13, depending on the race, you might swim 200 or 300 meters, bike 10 or 15 kilometers, and run 2 or 3 kilometers. So in order to swim 200 meters in a 25 meter pool, you would swim back and forth 4 times.

Once you enter races at the 14 to 15 year age group you might be doing the race for fun if you are new to the sport or you can compete in regional championships if you decide to be competitive. At these ages use of more technical biking equipment is normally allowed, including clipless pedals, aero-bars, and racing wheels, which are not allowed in the younger age groups for safety reasons. At this age your races' distances would be around a 300-500 meter swim, 15 kilometer bike, and a 3 or 4 kilometer run, depending on each individual event.

At ages 16 to 19 you can still race just to have fun, but potentially can compete in National Championships if you do well and choose to be competitive.

Normally the standard distance for this age group is a 750 meter swim, a 20 kilometer bike, and a 5 kilometer run. If you decide to race with the best and do well you could eventually earn the right to compete at the National level and even represent Canada at the World Junior Sprint Championships. If you developed a passion for the sport and decided to be highly competitive, this could be a major step toward representing your country in the Olympic Games.

The Olympic distance triathlon is a 1.5 kilometer swim, a 40 kilometer bike, and a 10 kilometer run.

Once you are 18 you can compete in pretty well any triathlon in the world except for championship races or the Olympics as an age-grouper and still be entering for fun and at no time do you have to be racing to win unless you want to.

The best part about triathlon is that it's not necessary to spend tons of money on equipment and you can take time to decide if you want to keep doing it for fun or if you want to become competitive. When you first enter the world of triathlon, the main emphasis is on fun, safety, developing new skills, and becoming healthy and fit.

Just keep in mind that regardless if you are 6 years old or 75 years old, you can always be a triathlete for fun and never have to worry about competing if you don't want to. There is nothing that requires you to have a perfect body or to be a super athlete. All you really need is to believe in yourself and have a desire to achieve a better level of fitness and health.

I think it's the perfect sport for having fun, learning new skills, meeting new people, and getting super fit.

If you live in Canada, you can get information about triathlons for youth at http://triathloncanada.com.

If you live in the United Kingdom, there is an excellent series of triathlons for kids 8-13 years old called "Corus Kids of Steel Triathlon." You can find information here: http://corustriathlon.com

There are also kids' triathlons all through the United States. They can be found simply by searching by the state you are interested in. For instance type "California Kids Triathlons" or "Oregon kids triathlons" into your computer search engine and that will lead you to all the available kids' races in that state. There are some *huge* kids' races in California, because triathlon has become so popular.

So realistically, you could even go in races in other countries if you happen to be there on holidays with your parents. Most races are open to kids from everywhere.

As I mentioned in the beginning of the chapter, triathlon is one of the fastest growing sports in the world. It's an excellent choice for fitness and for getting yourself out there and feeling what it's like when your body is functioning at peak efficiency as you get fitter and fitter. Triathlon may be the catalyst that will lead you to another sport that you may find you love. For instance, maybe you will embrace swimming or running as your sport, or possibly your newfound fitness and confidence will enable you to make that team you always wanted to be a part of.

If you combine sports and fitness with a healthy and nutritious diet you will see remarkable changes in how you look and feel, but more than that, it will instill a new sense of confidence and self-esteem you will carry with you for the rest of your life.

Chapter Fifteen

* SWIM, BIKE, RUN *

If you can already swim, you are well on your way to becoming a triathlete. However, there's a good chance you can't swim, and possibly you're even a little afraid of the water. There's nothing wrong with that. Being a bit afraid instills a healthy respect for the water, and that's a good thing.

When I saw my first triathlon almost 25 years ago, I just knew I had to cross that finish line. At the time, I was watching the Hawaii Ironman Triathlon on Television. I had no idea what it was, but it intrigued me and almost seemed to be calling out to me. I was 33 years old and a runner, but had a fear of water over my head and couldn't swim a single stroke. However I made up my mind that I was going to learn to swim and compete in the Hawaii Ironman one day soon.

I took kids' lessons for adults and soon for the very first time I was able to swim from one side of the pool to the other. Yes, I mean the other *side*. It took a while before I could swim to the other *end*. In the following months I swam every chance I had until finally after about six months I could swim almost the entire Ironman swim distance of 3.8 kilometers in the pool. It was that day that I realized I was going to enter the Ironman triathlon in Kona, Hawaii.

It you look at the back cover of this book, you will see the picture of me crossing that same finish line I had seen on television just two years earlier. Yes, I survived the 3.8 kilometer Ironman swim and finished the 180 km bike and 42.2 km run as well and over 14 hours later became an Ironman.

That single moment in time when I crossed the finish line changed my life forever.

So believe in yourself and have confidence that you can learn how to swim if you persist and don't give up on yourself. If possible it's best to have expert, qualified swimming instruction to get you started. Once you learn the technique of proper swimming, it's simply a matter of working at it, and over time you will get more comfortable in the water. Once you have learned the proper technique, go swimming with your parents or friends, and always swim where there is a lifeguard watching over you. Even the best of swimmers should never really swim alone in areas where there is nobody to look out for them. Safety should always be your number one concern when you are in or near the water.

The key thing I learned over the years about swimming when it comes to triathlons is to develop a long, smooth stroke. When you reach the point that you are able to swim laps in a pool, concentrate on *how* you get to the other end of the pool, not *how fast* you get there. Learn to glide more and take fewer and fewer strokes. As you continue on in the sport of triathlon, you will soon realize that the more energy you save in the swim, the better you will feel in the bike and run. This is especially true as the distances you swim, bike and run get longer and longer.

If you are just learning how to swim, you should make a point of trying to swim several times a week so your body can get used to it. Your muscles have a memory and can remember the actions it takes to complete your swim stroke and will tend to repeat it over and over. That's why it's important to learn properly from the very beginning. If you learn poor technique, that's the technique your muscles will be repeating over and over again. It's very hard to break bad swimming habits. Certainly it can be done, but the best way is to learn proper swimming skills from the very beginning.

There are so many adults who can't swim. They just never took the time or had the opportunity to learn when they were young. Don't let that happen to you. Being able to swim can very well save your life one day, or possibly enable you to save someone else who is in trouble in the water. It's also one of the best sports there is for fitness.

If you decide to become a triathlete and enter a race, be sure to check out the distance you will be swimming in your event. As I mentioned earlier, it will depend on your age. That is the distance you want to get used to doing in the pool once you have learned the basics of how to swim.

BIKE

Most likely you know how to bike, but don't get out on your bike that often. If that's the case, try and bike a few days a week to get your body used to it. If you already bike quite a bit, then you most likely will just have to work on the distances you are biking. Once again, check to see how far you will be biking in the triathlon you plan to enter. Work on things like biking in a nice straight line and having a nice comfortable "spin." As you take part in your first triathlons don't worry so much about how fast you go. Enjoy the event and have fun and start to get used to how it feels to bike on the road with others around you and how good it feels to be in motion and part of something special.

Feel the action of your legs as they travel in a circle, see the sun glint off the shiny spokes of your bike and hear the hum of your tires as they skim across the road.

It truly is good to be alive and active and fit.

RUN

Maybe for you running comes easy. Or maybe you are overweight and running is something you feel is beyond you. After running just a few meters you are breathing heavy and might even feel a bit dizzy. Most likely it's because your heart has to work so hard to accomplish what you are asking of it. Maybe to this point in your life you have had really poor eating habits and have neglected your fitness.

Well, that was then and this is now. All things are possible if it's in your heart to make a change for the better.

All I could manage when I first started to run some 32 years ago was about twice around the inside of a gym. I had decided I wanted to run a marathon. However, I had smoked for almost 15 years and this was a sudden change for my body to absorb. It was that first day that I ran that convinced me that smoking had to become something in my past. I gave up smoking and began my journey to the finish line of my first marathon. I ran inside for weeks because I was to embarrassed to run outside. I felt somehow inadequate and had this feeling that I didn't belong out there.

I was wrong.

I persisted in my running, and every week I started to breathe better and feel better. One day I ran 120 laps around the inside of that gym. I remember thinking "this is crazy. I can't run around these corners anymore." So I took it outside.

For weeks I ran and I ran and I ran. As the weeks passed, I ran further and further. Forty minutes, an hour, ninety minutes and then two hours.

In less than a year I crossed the finish line of my first marathon in 3 hours and twenty eight minutes. I have not smoked a cigarette since. I have run over 35 marathons, a couple of 80 kilometer races and have been entered in 14 Ironman triathlons.

The only thing that brought me from being an out of shape, smoking couch potato to where I am today, was not quitting after those very first two laps that I ran. Had I quit at that moment, I never would have become a runner, and I never would have been tempted to take on the Ironman, so I would never have learned how to swim.

I can't even imagine what direction my life would have taken had I carried on the way I was going.

You have the power to begin now. You have such a big future ahead of you. A future so full of possibilities. Don't feel for a minute that you don't belong out on the bike path or on a treadmill, or along the side of the road running. When I am out running and see someone who is obviously overweight but out there trying, I have nothing but respect and admiration for them.

If you are new to running and have weight to lose and fitness to gain, begin by walking. Walk for 20 minutes 4 or 5 times and then walk for 30 minutes 4 or 5 times. Keep building until you can walk for an hour. Try and walk at least 3 times a week so your body can get used to it. You might be sore for a while, but that is just your body getting accustomed to something new you are demanding of it.

Once you can walk for an hour adjust your workout. Walk for 10 minutes then walk *fast* (power-walk) for 5 minutes. Repeat that at least twice and then end your workout with walking at an easy pace. At this point you can progress according to how you feel. You can try doing the 10 minutes easy and 5 minutes hard sequence 3 or 4 times.

Then you can try walking easy for 5 minutes and walking fast for 10 minutes and keep building on that. Take the time you need. Don't rush it. So what if it takes two years to get to your first triathlon? You have your whole life in front of you.

One day you will be ready to try a 5 minute easy walk warm-up and then "power-walk" for 20 minutes straight and then end with a 5 minute easy cool-down walk.

Build on that.

If you are combining a new, healthy diet with your new found fitness plan, you will begin to feel and look better than you ever thought possible.

Don't give up. It took years to get where you are and it will take time to change the rhythm of your life, but it will happen if it's in your heart to make a change.

When you feel you are ready, (even if it takes months) do a 5 minute easy walk to warm up, power walk for 15 minutes, and then run slowly for 5 minutes. If it feels okay, do it twice. Then build on that.

When that feels okay, do a 5 minute easy walk to warm up, and then run easily for 10 minutes, and if it feels good keep running and make it 15.

Hey. Wow! Guess what? You're running! You're on your way and you can progress at your own speed and take it as far as you want. The message I'm trying to give you is that even the longest journey begins with a single step.

That's what I meant at the very beginning of this book when I said that you are truly magnificent. We all are. It's just that so many of us just don't realize it. Regardless of where your life has brought you to this point in time, there will always be a sparkling gem within you just waiting for a chance to shine.

Swim, bike, and run.

Embrace fitness as a way of life and choose the best possible nutrition to fuel your body and one day you will be in awe of the power you have within you.

Chapter Sixteen

* WHERE DO I BEGIN? *

It may be that the information in this book overwhelms you a bit. Maybe you have learned things about nutrition and food in general that you never realized before. Maybe you have never considered, or perhaps given up on the idea that you could ever be an athlete of any sort and yet, I believe you can.

Maybe you are already fit and athletic and eat a healthy diet. If you do, you deserve a lot of credit and good for you!

Chances are, though, if you are reading this book, you are at a point in your life where it's time to take control and make some positive changes in the direction life is taking you.

The world is full of good intentions. It's full of people who set their minds on getting fitter, healthier, and simply doing things better. Many however lose sight of their goal soon after they begin and eventually fall back into their old ways.

Why?

Maybe because they don't see results right away. Maybe because their muscles get sore and ache when they try and become physically active. Maybe the addictive nature of sugar and fat laden fast foods is difficult for them to fight.

Maybe it's just too hard and it's easier to promise themselves they will try again next month or next year or "some other time."

Maybe it's because they're well into adulthood and have spent so many years living an unhealthy way of life, that it gets harder and harder with each passing year to try and change the way things are so they simply don't bother.

That doesn't have to be the way it is for you.

Say for example you are 15 years old and the culmination of

your life has brought you from the miracle of birth to where you are this very second as you read this sentence.

You came into this world in a state of near perfection and like a book full of blank pages, your story had yet to be written.

Your physical image, how you think, and how people perceive you are a culmination of what you have done with your life since the second you opened your eyes for the very first time.

So what have **you** done with your gift of life? What have you become? What do you see when you look in the mirror? Who do you blame for the way things are?

Do you smoke, drink, do drugs, eat crappy food, bully others, let yourself be bullied, spend too much time on the computer, cheat, steal, or do far worse in school than you are really capable of? In short, is your life going in a direction that you are not particularly proud of and would like to make some changes but don't know where to begin?

Well if you have read this far into <u>Lifestruck</u>, you are on your way, and the opportunity for change that might well alter the course of your life is upon you.

Start now, start easy, and slowly ease yourself into a completely new way of life.

Remember that it's taken years to get to where you are today, and it will take patience, effort, and self-belief to unearth the remarkable person and miracle of creation that lives inside you just waiting to come out into the light.

Start by looking back at what got you to where you are now. Look back over the last year and think about the way you have chosen to nourish your body. What have you been eating? What have you been doing? Smoking, drinking, drugs? All this goes into your body and has played a role in the make-up of who you are right now.

Here is how you begin.

Start slowly, but always move forward. Once you decide in your heart to take the first step on your journey of self-discovery and to embrace "a better way", always move forward and don't look back. What *has* happened is done. What **will** happen begins in the moment that is in front of you right this instant.

Every time you eat something, stop for just a second and consider that this is the fuel that will propel you, and go a long way toward defining who you are, how you feel, and the body image you project. Good nutrition has the amazing power to change life as you know it.

Slowly begin to eliminate foods from your diet that you now know are not really that good for you. Instead, substitute these unhealthy foods with some of the really great food choices you now realize are good for you.

Just like the kids who grew up on the farm, embrace wholesome, healthy food as a way of life and start to look at the unhealthy choices like bags of chips, chocolate, soft drinks, processed foods, and fast foods as very occasional treats.

It's almost like your entire generation feels there is no way they can change what is. Like I said earlier it's not all your fault because you are a product of the environment you were born into and are under the impression that because this is the way things are, you are stuck with it. However, you have the power to break away and take your own path and control your own destiny and not let others dictate your future.

You will start to notice things as you begin to eat healthier. You will sleep better, have more energy, and simply start looking healthier. You will even start doing better in school. You will become more confident and people will be drawn to you and you will most likely have more friends.

At the same time as you adjust your nutrition habits, slowly begin your life of fitness. Ease yourself into a new, healthier way of life. Your first impulse might be to wake up in the morning and make a 100% change in your life and hit the ground running. This works for some people, but being too impetuous might be asking too much of your body too soon and it will rebel.

That's what happens to adults when they push too hard too soon looking for that "quick fix" and their muscles rebel at these sudden demands. Remember that you are the boss. Your body is a miracle of genetic engineering and will respond to the positive changes you are making. Give it time to do it's work. Once it realizes that you expect it to power you through your newfound realm of fitness, it will begin to make the necessary adjustments.

That's exactly why I suggested a non-runner and a person just starting out on a healthier way of life begin slowly by walking, walking faster, and then slowly running over weeks and even months. Using this format in whatever fitness activity you do will give your body time to adapt. Just remember, move forward, always forward and change will happen.

Your heart will strengthen in order to pump life-giving blood to all those muscles you are working. Your veins will become unclogged and you will lose unneeded weight as you eliminate unhealthy foods from your diet and introduce new, healthy "power" food that will fuel the high performance engine that is the new you. The quality fat you eat will create the fuel that powers you and the healthy complex carbohydrates will create the fire to burn the fat. The protein you eat will help rebuild and strengthen your muscles, bones, heart, and tone your entire body as it becomes accustomed to your new and better way of life.

Do this for a year you would see remarkable changes. You will be so impressed by those changes that it will move you to look at life differently. It will give you a glimpse of the power you have within you to go any direction you want. It will be a lifestyle you will want to adopt forever.

So where do you begin?

You begin by embracing the idea that there is "a better way" for you. There is a better way to live your life that will open doors that you may have thought were closed to you forever.

Chapter Seventeen

* BALANCE *

The key to success in your school years is to develop *balance* in your life.

It's great to do well in all your school work and have top marks. It's also great to maintain your health and a high level of fitness. However, to concentrate all your efforts in just one direction will leave you lacking in the areas you ignore.

That's the reason why schools are structured the way they are and exactly why they offer athletics and other extra-curricular activities as well as academics. It's essential to exercise both your body and mind because ultimately the strength you build in both these areas will provide the balanced foundation for your journey into adulthood.

It's hard to have much self-esteem and the will to excel if you have no family structure, no self-confidence, and a lack of belief in yourself. It doesn't have to be like that. No matter what twists and turns life has thrown at you, you have the power within you to take a new direction.

Strive for balance in all things.

How often have you heard the word "moderation"? Well, there's a good reason why the word is used all the time. It seems that as soon as something is overdone it begins to create problems. If you have a chocolate or two from the box, it's not so bad, but if you eat the whole box, it's not so great. There are dozens of other food choices that most likely have the phrase "okay to eat in moderation" in their description somewhere.

If you get a bit of sun, it's good for you, but stay out there too long and you will most likely burn and be in a world of pain for a while and be at risk from those dreaded UV rays. On the other hand, if you never go outside you will deprive yourself of that healthy glow and sense of well-being that sun and fresh air provide.

Sacrificing your social life and physical fitness in order to spend every waking hour buried in school work makes about as much sense as quitting school in grade ten so you can go to hockey camps or play on a junior team somewhere with the hopes of one day being a pro prospect. That's exactly why most colleges in the U.S. require athletes to have a certain grade average before they can be part of a team. Ignoring your fitness in order to excel at academics is as counter-productive as giving everything to a sport and ignoring your education. That's why schools are all about balance. In order to make it in this world, it's to your benefit to be a well-rounded individual.

There is no way I would ever suggest to anyone they train for eight hours a day to be a triathlete. That makes about as much sense as spending three hours a day on a cell phone and another 6 hours a day on a computer, yet that's exactly what happens far too often.

Think balance.

Exercise your mind and exercise your body. Spend time with cool friends and spend time with family. Spend quality time with others and spend quality time with yourself. Be comfortable in groups and be comfortable with the one you are with when you are alone.

> Work hard. Play hard.

> Love others. Love yourself.

> Spend time with nature. Go shopping.

> Help others. Let others help you.

> Be proud. Be humble.

> Be cautious. Be adventurous.

> Get excited. Remain calm.

Life is all about balance.

I once met a girl who could speak five languages, run like the wind, was a skilled scuba diver, looked awesome in a bikini, managed a pharmacy, and could cook the lights out. She could also tell great jokes and walk across the room with three big books on her head. Now *that's* balance! However, what stood out the most was her love of life and how she was never afraid to try something new. She was never afraid to challenge herself. She never accepted that she just *couldn't* do something. It never bothered her if she couldn't do something *well*, but it would have really bothered her if she never tried. That was her secret.

One day she wrote to me from her country and said she had cancer. She fought and won the battle of her life and she later told me that as she lay dying and fought to live, she reached a point where she felt she was teetering on a fence. If she fell one way she would die, and if she fell the other way she would live.

She told me she was convinced the difference between her living or dying was the health, fitness, and strength that she took into battle. That, she said, along with her love of life and will to live, made all the difference. Don't ever underestimate the power of balance.

For some reason I have always remembered a line from Sinbad the Sailor by Ulysses S. Grant.

"I am a part of all that I have met."

That one line has so much truth to it. Everything you do, everything you experience, and everything and everyone you cross paths with in your journey of life will become a part of who you are.

I read once how most people in the world only use a small percentage of their mental and physical capacity. I think one of the reasons is probably because we allow ourselves to become too one-dimensional. When we are young and in the formative years we are too quick to accept our situation and adopt the attitude that things are what they are and will never change. We can't make the team, so it means we will never be athletic. We aren't "A" students so it means we will never be smart.

Take control of your life and challenge yourself to improve on every level. You will soon discover strength and ability inside you that you never knew existed. There is no reason you have to accept your lot in life. We can't all have perfect families. We can't all have all the material things that money can buy. Things just happen in life, but there is no reason you have to roll over and accept it. Take control. It's your life. Take responsibility. There is no magic age or time to wait for. Are you 10, 12, 14, 16? What are you waiting for? It's your life and it's within you to make positive changes.

Take action and look for that balance.

If you can't make the team, so what? Build your health and build your strength. When you see the change in your body, you will feel the change in your mind. Your self-doubt will become self-esteem. You will be on the inside *doing* and not on the outside *looking in*. Once you get the ball rolling and become more self-confident with who you have become, all aspects of your life will improve.

Chapter Eighteen

* TRIATHLON ... A FAMILY AFFAIR *

As triathlon grows, so do the number of families that participate in the sport together. I was once in an Ironman triathlon that had three generations of the same family entered in the race.

There were a daughter, a mother, and a grandfather all competing in one of the most challenging endurance races in the world. How cool is that? Triathlon truly is a sport for everyone.

It must be so special to share a common goal and to learn from each other. How can it not help but create a strong family bond? This is the story of one of those amazing triathlon families who share a lifestyle of healthy eating and fitness that best describe what <u>Lifestruck</u> is all about.

TRIATHLON AS A FAMILY SPORT

Heather MacCollum – Mom. 34 years old, four boys later, and still running.

Robert MacCollum – Dad. 34 years old, four boys later, and still fast on the bike. Previous history of road racing for 10 years.

Kain MacCollum – the eldest. 13 years old, Kamloops track and field team. Kain enjoys the bike, but excels in the run. The swim is a technical difficulty to be overcome, which he acknowledges has not come naturally and is something he has to work at.

Caydon MacCollum – next in line. 8 years old, loves the bike, great endurance. Loves to practice, dislikes the spectators. Needs more confidence to race.

Kellen MacCollum – next after Caydon. 6 years old, learning

to bike, likes to run. Just wanting to keep up whatever way possible. Determination at its best.

Cadel MacCollum – The baby. 20 months old. Just keep me moving one way or another and I will be happy; stop and I will scream. Excels in running and swimming, really wants to bike but cannot reach the pedals.

We all have our strengths. We all have our weaknesses; that is why triathlon is so great for the family. It combines everyone's strengths, weaknesses, likes and dislikes. You are always leaning new things from each other and the people around you.

Some of us love to run, like to swim, and can bike (that is Mom). As a family we have learned to do all the sports together. When we run, Mom, Dad and Kain run, Caydon rides his bike, and Kellen and Cadel ride in the double chariot. Sometimes we combine walks with runs, and everyone runs. We even made up a park workout and use park benches for dips, push-ups and planks.

The road bike is a little more complicated and took some fine tuning. Because the youngest three are too little to bike on the big roads, they ride in the van, movies, books and sightseeing along with cheering on the riders. Mom is a photographer, so she is always up for a great cycling picture. Many times Dad drives while Mom and Kain ride one direction and Dad bikes it back. He is faster so he usually beats us all home. Most often Dad rides to family destinations. If we go to the lake for the day, Dad rides while the rest of us follow a bit behind. We all get there at the same time and then play for the day or take turns open water swimming while the youngest play at the edge or in the kayak.

The open water swim has taken the purchase of a double Kayak. While Mom and Kain or Dad and Kain swim, the little ones ride along in the Kayak. They love the water and practice paddling, cheering and sightseeing. It is amazing when we look back at how much the younger three have learned just by being with us while we are training and how much we value their encouragement. They have fallen in love with triathlons by just watching and being part of it.

The boys have become very aware that what we put in our mouths is our fuel. It gives us the energy and drive for what we are to do with our bodies. Kain is very concerned about his pre-race fuel and protein intake. He has learned so much from asking questions and talking with other athletic trainers. The other boys have come to the conclusion that Fruit Loops do not make your day run better. We have tried to keep a low sugar (no refined sugar) and a daily healthy diet. Breakfast being the most important, consists of the day's start. We try to have healthy pancakes, eggs and toast (five dozen a week) or fruity French toast, no syrup involved. The boys have quickly adapted to the full breakfast and enjoy it every day.

Triathlon has given the boys an understanding of new sports, cross training, being the best you can be even if it is not your favorite. Because of the different aspects of Triathlons you never get bored; you are always changing it up a little.

Kain has excelled in school. We feel that his athletic abilities have given him confidence and a drive to excel in the classroom as well as on the course. He has met so many great kids involved with sports who love to go for bike rides or a run instead of sitting in front of electronics. The Kids of Steel is encouraging and exciting as so many ages race to finish three fun sports all in a short period of time.

There is no better feeling in the world than to cross the finish line and see your family, training partners and competitors all in one cheering you on! Whether or not you are good at only one part of triathlon or good at them all, they complement each other, making you faster, stronger and fitter in all sports.

Chapter Nineteen

* WHAT WILL I BE? *

This is a question that has plagued and mystified young adults for generation after generation. From the time you are old enough to reason you most likely started thinking about "what will I be when I grow up?" In your mind's eye you were a cowboy, a doctor, a nurse, an astronaut, or a great athlete. Maybe you even dressed up like them and pretended you were them.

It's not uncommon at all for students to leave high school and begin College or University and still not know "what they want to be."

I'm a great example of that.

My father was a baker for a supermarket when I was in grade 11 and looking for a part-time job, so he got me a job in that store.

After grade 12 I left home and never had the opportunity to go to College or University. Instead I decided to join the work-force. The only place I had any experience was (you guessed it) the grocery business, so that's where I applied and that's where I was hired full-time.

I'm 59 now and in my fortieth year with that same retail grocery company.

When I was 56 I realized what I wanted to be when I grew up. I wanted to be an author and have the ability to write something that was motivational and inspirational enough that it would help others improve their lives.

As a result my first book, Ironstruck, was born and still I get emails from around the world that go something like this. "Until I read your book, I never knew what I was capable of. I quit smoking, got fit, and a year later did an Ironman Triathlon. Thank you, it has changed my life."

I could think to myself, "I wasted so many years," but in reality

I would sooner take the high road and to be honest, I'm so grateful I came to the realization when I did and was given the opportunity to reach out to others, like I am reaching out to you, and perhaps helping you realize there indeed is "a better way."

However, it does mystify me how I let so many years pass, because even back in high school, literature was my favorite subject, and I loved to read and write. I had the passion for writing in my heart, but never acted on it and ignored all the clues. Don't let this happen to you.

Just think of the advantage you will have if you realize early on in the high school years exactly what you want to do with your future. How amazing would it be if you had a passion for something early in life and could put all your energy toward being successful at it long after you left high school?

You are indeed the future of the world as we know it.

In your city, your country, your continent and all over the world there are others students sitting at a desk just like yours who will one day shape the future of the world. Future Presidents and Prime Ministers, doctors, scientists, teachers, and astronauts are all sitting at a desk just like you are. They have families, friends, bad days and good days, and are really no different than you.

Except for maybe one or two things.

They have vision and most likely a passion for something and are able to put the two together and set their sights on a goal that goes way beyond high school. It is such a gift to come to this realization and actually run with it and see it through to the end.

I knew such a person in high school. From the time he was about 10 years old, he built model planes and had dreams of flying jet planes. Once he had a direction he wanted his life to go he was able to chart his path and do all the right things and take all the right classes in University. He went into Air Cadets and then the Air Reserve and took courses that would enhance his chances of actually realizing his dream.

Fifteen years ago he retired as a major in the Air , and indeed, he did fly in the jets he used to dream of.

So, search your heart. What do you have a passion for? Do you have a love for animals and their well-being? Maybe being a veterinarian is in your future. Do you have a passion for words and the ability to make your thoughts flow? You could be a great author. Do you look at the world around you or possibly your country and the way it is headed and believe you could do a better job of things? You could be the leader of your country, and along with other great leaders of the world, chart the course humanity will take into the 22nd century.

The opportunity is there for the taking. There is a student just like you going to high school somewhere in your country who will be filling that role one day. Why not you? Someone is going to do it.

Learn all you can about the politics of your country and chart your course through University or College that will help and enter the political arena and begin your journey. Be a party volunteer and help the candidate of your choice and all the time, listen and learn until it becomes your turn to shine.

The whole point is, once you identify your true passion in life, focus on that goal. Every day, pay attention to things that intrigue you. Pay attention to things you do that amaze others, yet come as second nature to you.

I remember one kid in high school who could sketch amazing figures on paper. All you had to do was name an object or animal and his pencil would blur across the paper and like magic an amazing image would appear. I don't know what happened to him, but I hope he became a great artist or designer or something else worthy of such talent.

One thing I have noticed so many times in my journey through life is that so many people are born with so much and yet are able to achieve so little and then there are those incredible people who are born with so little yet fly with the eagles and are the great achievers of the world.

Which one are you? Either way you have the opportunity for greatness and the ability to achieve great things and help shape the world we live in and make it a better place for everyone.

You will be taking the first vital steps once you embrace a life of excellent nutrition and fitness that will be the cornerstone and catalyst for all the amazing possibilities the future has in store for you.

Chapter Twenty

Hopefully <u>Lifestruck</u> will inspire you to attain a higher level of health and fitness. If it has, then you are well on your way to witnessing a transformation to a "new you" and will discover potential within yourself you never knew existed.

By embracing a healthier way of living on a day to day basis, changes in how you look, feel and perform will manifest themselves in many ways. At first these changes will be subtle as your body gradually adjusts to the changes you are making in the way you live your life.

It won't be long before you begin to feel better and sleep better. Over time you will begin to notice obvious physical changes. You will boost your immune system and as a result be better prepared to ward off, or at the very least diminish, the effects of common ailments like colds and the 'flu. Unneeded fat will slowly begin to melt away, and your muscles will take on more definition. Improved blood circulation through fitness and eating the best possible foods will make your hair shine and your eyes lively and bright. Your complexion will take on a healthy glow. Physically, you will soon be able to do twice as much with half the effort.

And that's just the physical changes.

Embracing a healthier way of life will also boost your confidence and self-esteem to new heights as you see more and more changes begin to take place in how you look and feel. You will do better scholastically in school and the aura of success and confidence you exude will attract others to you and you your social life will improve dramatically. Maybe triathlon will be the catalyst for finding another sport that is just right for you. Lance Amstrong was a triathlete at one time and look at him now. He has won the hardest bike race in the world over and over again. As much as you might not think so now, you could go on to be a world class athlete one day.

As you embrace your new way of living and begin to make your way in the world, always be aware of those around you.

Watch out for those who seem shy, afraid, and are desperately in need of encouragement, direction, and friendship. They won't be hard to spot, because they may remind you of yourself before you had the courage and knowledge to take control of your life.

Help them. Encourage them. Stick up for the bullied and downtrodden. Yes there are bad people in the world, but always remember that there are many, many more good people. Be one of the good people and help lost souls where you can. Often those who lose their way in life are those same kids who fell through the cracks in school. By reaching out in some small way you could change the course of their lives for the better and as result make the world a better place for everyone. It might be as simple as giving them a copy of Lifestruck to read.

When the final tally of your life is taken and what you did with the time you spent on this earth is set out before you, remember that what you leave behind in the world is worth a lot more than what you take from it.

The medals and trophies on my wall bring back echoes of past glory and unforgettable moments in my life, but still, I've come to the realization that life is not always deemed a success by the medals on your wall, but rather the ones you inspire others to put on theirs.

END

MORE FROM THE AUTHOR

➢ Ironstruck.ca.

➢ Lifestruck.ca (coming soon).

➢ http://www.lulu.com/content/543252 – Ironstruck...The
Ironman Triathlon Journey.

➢ http://www.lulu.com/content/3227806 – Ironstruck? 500
Ironman Triathlon Questions and Answers.

LaVergne, TN USA
19 March 2011

220754LV00001B/7/P